FOUNDATIONS OF DISTINCTIVE FEATURE THEORY

FOUNDATIONS OF DISTINCTIVE FEATURE THEORY

Christiane A. M. Baltaxe, Ph.D

Assistant Professor of Psychiatry
and Behavioral Sciences
Neuropsychiatric Institute
The Center for the
Health Sciences
University of California
at Los Angeles

University Park Press
Baltimore

UNIVERSITY PARK PRESS
International Publishers in Science and Medicine
233 East Redwood Street
Baltimore, Maryland 21202

Copyright © 1978 by University Park Press

Typeset by Everybodys Press.
Manufactured in the United States of America by
The Maple Press Company.

Library of Congress Cataloging in Publication Data

Baltaxe, Christiane A. M.
Foundations of distinctive feature theory.

Bibliography: p.
Includes index.
1. Distinctive features (linguistics) 2. Linguistics—History—20th
century. I. Title. [DNLM: 1. Language development. 2. Phonetics.
3. Speech—Physiology. P215 B197f]
P218 B3   414   78-1520
ISBN 0-8391-1212-2

to Mutti, Stephanie, Robin, Michael, and especially George

CONTENTS

FOREWORD

The hypothesis that the large phonemic inventory of any language can be described by a smaller set of distinctive features has received widespread acceptance in recent years. This acceptance is well justified on both theoretical and empirical grounds. The distinctive feature concept has been incorporated into linguistic theories: sound change, morphophonemic variation, and phonological systems. Experimental psychology has furnished support for the reality of distinctive features in studies of short-term memory, errors in perception, and psychophysical scaling. Moreover, the distinctive feature concept is proving to be a powerful tool in "applied" areas such as speech pathology and automated speech recognition. Distinctive feature analyses in studies of language acquisition and deviant speech are now commonplace.

As evidence accumulates to support the distinctive feature approach in general, we need to bear in mind that there are still significant issues that remain unresolved. Is there a universal set of distinctive features? Is there a universal feature hierarchy? Are all features binary, or are some multivalued or even continuous? Are the features orthogonal? Which is the optimal level(s) for specifying the features (articulatory, acoustic, perceptual, other)? These and other important questions are still open to debate. People who apply distinctive feature theory in their clinical or research areas need to be aware that any particular feature system is not *the* feature system, that each feature system represents one theoretical interpretation of the distinctive feature concept. Depending on the underlying theoretical assumptions, a feature system may or may not be suitable for a specific application.

Clearly, the user of a distinctive feature system should understand its theoretical foundations. However, much of the source material for theoretical understanding has not been readily available. This volume, by Christiane Baltaxe, helps to fill this gap. It is an exhaustive treatise on the historical foundations of distinctive feature theory. It discusses the origins of the distinctive feature concept in the Prague School of linguistics, the evolution of the theory, and the divergence in the views of the two co-founders of distinctive feature theory, Trubetzkoy and Jakobson. In the United States, we have been exposed primarily to the Jakobsonian interpretation of distinctive feature theory. This approach was presented initially in *Preliminaries to Speech Analysis* (Jakobson, Fant, and Halle, 1952) and has been incorporated with modifications into the phonological component of generative grammar (see Chomsky and Halle, *The Sound Patterns of English,* 1968). Trubetzkoy's approach to distinctive features has been neglected in the United States in part because his work has not been available in English until recently. Dr. Baltaxe has already greatly contributed to our understanding of Trubetzkoy's work by her publication of the first English translation (1969) of Trubetzkoy's *Principles of Phonology* (1939). The present volume complements this earlier work by elucidating the theoretical issues and placing them in historical context.

Foundations of Distinctive Feature Theory provides a sound basis for continuing our research and application with the awareness that distinctive feature theory is still being developed. Those who apply distinctive features in their analyses of phonemes in clinical work, education, engineering, psychology, language studies, and other fields are not only making use of a powerful tool but are also involved in testing the theory, answering some of the unresolved questions, and furthering the historical development of distinctive feature theory. A thorough reading of this book leads to an understanding of the fundamental issues involved in a distinctive feature theory.

Sadanand Singh, Ph.D.
Professor
Speech and Hearing Institute
The University of Texas
Health Science Center
Houston, Texas

ACKNOWLEDGMENTS

I would like to thank Jaan Puhvel for his support throughout the research which forms the basis for this book. I am indebted to Peter Ladefoged for his helpful comments. Roman Jakobson has clarified for me some points of difference between himself and N. S. Trubetzkoy in the development of phonological theory. Alexander Isačenko has contributed in terms of "eyewitness" accounts of Prague School development. I would also like to thank Henrik Birnbaum, Dean Worth, and William Bright for helpful comments and reading parts of the manuscript. I am especially grateful for many hours of fruitful discussion with Pavle Ivič.

Thanks are also due James Q. Simmons, III, and Sadanand Singh for the encouragement they gave me to complete the manuscript. Dorothy Disterheft was very helpful in assisting with the typing and proofing of the manuscript. My special thanks go to George Baltaxe and Stephanie, Robin, and Michael for their understanding and consideration.

INTRODUCTION

The development of distinctive feature theory in the United States has been associated primarily with the name of Roman Jakobson and the work which he wrote in English. There can be no doubt that the main impetus to feature analysis in the United States derived from Jakobson's two now classic works, *Preliminaries to Speech Analysis* (1952) written with Gunnar Fant and Morris Halle, and *Fundamentals of Language* (1956), in which Jakobson collaborated with Halle. It would be wrong to claim, however, that the origin of feature theory rested on the sudden and brilliant flash of insight of one man alone. On the contrary, the roots of distinctive feature theory are buried deep in Prague School phonology. Another early phonologist, Nikolai Sergevič Trubetzkoy, figures centrally in its development. Distinctive feature theory represents the culmination of long years of phonological theorizing and practical work in typological studies and synchronic analysis of a wide range of languages. Interest in fields such as poetics may have helped direct attention to the prosodic characteristics of language and give impetus to the subsequent development of a system of prosodic features.

The concept of the distinctive feature only gradually ripened in Prague phonology, and the Jakobsonian distinctive features of *Preliminaries* and *Fundamentals* represent a direct continuation of that development.

Since the feature concept arose in the ambience of European linguistic studies, the original term to denote *feature* was the German *distinktive* or *phonologisch relevante Eigenschaft* ("distinctive" or "phonologically relevant property"). The term *Unterscheidungsmerkmal* ("differential mark or property") can also be found. After Jakobson came to the United States, he adopted the term *distinctive feature* from Bloomfield's *Language* (1933). However, Bloomfield had used the term in the sense of phoneme (p. 77ff.).

As is known, Jakobson's contributions to linguistics cover a wide and varied area of interest, and many of his insights and hypotheses have provided others with the incentive for further research. A trenchant analysis of Jakobson's contribution to the development of phonology in particular has been made by Ivić (1965b) in his exposition, "Roman Jakobson and the Growth of Phonology." Although Jakobson is seen today in the United States as the prime originator of distinctive feature theory and as the principal exponent of Prague phonology, the other central figure in the development of distinctive features and associated concepts—Nikolai Sergevič Trubetzkoy—is no less important. Trubetzkoy, whose linguistic genius rivaled that of Jakobson, had become fascinated by typological studies of a wide range of languages. He was rediscovered by Chomsky and Halle in their book, *The Sound Pattern of English* (1968), where the value of his theories and practical work in languages was accorded proper recognition. The earlier oversight can probably be explained by the relative inaccessibility of Trubetzkoy's works to English readers since they had been written in languages other than English. A translation of his compendium of phonological investigations, *Grundzüge der Phonologie* (1939), originally published in German, is now also available in English (Baltaxe,

1969), in addition to an earlier French translation (by Cantineau; see Jakobson, 1949).

Feature theory, as it is known today, essentially represents the outgrowth of the intellectual and scientific interplay of ideas and practical work of these two scholars. Although often separated by geological distances, Trubetzkoy and Jakobson, who was six years his junior, were bound to each other by ties of close friendship and common linguistic interests. There is no doubt that each exerted a considerable influence on the other and that both profited richly from this association.

Trubetzkoy, in the course of his development, became more and more interested in recurrent phonological patterns and universally valid laws about language. Although Jakobson, the younger man, may have originally inspired the older, it was Trubetzkoy who appeared to have matured faster in the development of his theories. At the time of his death, with his *Grundzüge der Phonologie* essentially completed, Trubetzkoy took a lasting place at the head of the Prague patrimony of phonology.

Trubetzkoy and Jakobson had been members of the Prague Linguistic Circle since its inception in 1926. Both had been under the influence of the Russian school of Baudouin de Courtenay, Fortunatov, and Ščerba, and both had enthusiastically embraced the ideas of de Saussure. Even though Trubetzkoy as well as Jakobson criticized the definitions of the linguistic conceptualization of Baudouin de Courtenay and Ščerba as insufficient and inexact, they would readily concur that their own conceptions represented a continuation in development of the basic ideas of these earlier scholars.

At times, the length of time between the original statement of an idea and the development of that idea can be considerable. This had been the case with the concept of opposition which had been offered by de Saussure, who had used it, though inconsistently and without conceptual elaboration. However, the concept of opposition went on to become one of the most important and fundamental notions for Trubetzkoy and Jakobson and for Prague phonological theory. De Saussure's by now famous dictum, "that phonemes were above all contrastive, relative, and negative units," thus was to become most influential in Prague phonological development, first in developing a theory of oppositions, and second in radically separating phonetics from phonology. Phonetics was considered a natural science, merely auxiliary to linguistics proper. The concept of the opposition was, of course, most fruitful, but the idea of a strict separation of phonetics and phonology was not defendable and ultimately had to be abandoned, although it had brought some insights.

The influences which transformed the theories of Trubetzkoy and Jakobson also affected the Prague School at large. With its epithets of structuralism and functionalism it generally represented the confluence of the ideas of the Russian school of Baudouin de Courtenay and Ščerba on the one hand, and of de Saussure on the other. Prague phonology and the development of distinctive features then took their identity from the specific direction and combination of these influences.

One aim of this volume is to present a balanced view of Trubetzkoy's and Jakobson's contributions to the various aspects of feature development. Although it is not always easy to account for the relative importance of the contributions of these two central personages, or to represent an accurate chronological account of the development of their ideas in feature theory, the literature gives many indications. Their close intellectual and scientific association, and the breadth of their shared interests, are well attested by 196 letters from Trubetzkoy to Jakobson. These represent the survival of a voluminous correspondence that was carried on between the two scholars between 1920 and 1938, the year of Trubetzkoy's tragic death and Jakobson's flight from central Europe. These letters miraculously survived World War II and were edited and published in 1975 by Roman Jakobson. They were published in their original Russian form, and it is hoped that they will soon become available in translation for those who do not read Russian. Unfortunately, Jakobson's letters to Trubetzkoy did not survive the war.

Trubetzkoy's letters attest to the fervor which the small circle of early phonologists brought to their endeavors. These letters frequently astound the reader with the amount of carefully delineated phonological and theoretical detail. In effect, some could almost be regarded on the level of today's preprints soliciting comments to articles subsequently to be published. Above all, these letters bear ample testimony to the importance of the interplay of ideas between the two pioneering scholars. They are also of interest from the point of view of the creative process which took place in these early investigations and which led to the development of a theory of distinctive features. A construct was developed first, frequently still based on insufficient phonological data. After additional supportive phonological data had been gathered from actual languages, this construct was then elaborated and substantiated. Frequently, the actual publication of relevant studies then followed only after the passage of several years, when additional data had been gathered. It is of interest to note that, although the exchange of letters took place in Russian, most of the subsequent articles which had been discussed or alluded to in these letters were published in either German or French.*

In perspective, it seems clear that this intellectual and scientific exchange between the two scholars, documented by these letters and by published articles, was absolutely essential to the development of the theory of distinctive features as we know it today. Both, letters and articles, attest to the fact that in many instances the two scholars were quite aware of potential pitfalls and difficulties in their phonological conceptions which needed to be worked out.

As claimed earlier, current feature theory rested to a high degree on the intellectual and scientific association between Trubetzkoy and Jakobson. However, it must be remembered that Trubetzkoy's work came to an abrupt end.† Fortunately, Jakobson was able to continue in

---

*Whenever quotations from these articles appear in the text, they have been translated by the author. For readers who are interested in comparing these translations with the original, appropriate citations have been provided.

† Trubetzkoy had angina and suffered a heart attack after a Gestapo interrogation and search of his home. He worked on the manuscript of *Grundzüge* and brought it to practical completion in the hospital before he died.

the development of his theories. It should therefore also not be surprising that considerable differences emerge between Trubetzkoy's final feature system dating back to 1938 and that of Jakobson as represented by *Preliminaries* and *Fundamentals* of 1952 and 1956, respectively.

There is no question that Trubetzkoy's features, as ultimately formulated and represented in his *Grundzüge der Phonologie,* are more complex, both in conception and elaboration, that those of Jakobson in *Preliminaries* and *Fundamentals.* Jakobson's final theory, embracing the criteria of simplicity, economy, and generality, now seems almost too simple in view of all the complexities of language and of the insights gained by the careful study of additional phonological detail from a variety of languages. From the point of view of theorizing, it could be claimed that such a simplified model was needed to bring preliminary order into the chaos of observed facts. The validation of such a model then provided a challenge to further study. Inherent in the validation process is, of course, the possibility that the model itself must be altered or expanded to accommodate facts previously not considered or overlooked. A careful reading of the literature shows that a number of such facts and insights which have contributed to the expansions of current distinctive feature theory had already been recognized by Trubetzkoy and had contributed to the complexity of *Grundzüge.* Jakobson's feature theory provided the impetus for further research and therefore was instrumental in the rediscovery of old facts and the discovery of new insights. The current revamped feature system of the Chomsky-Halle *Sound Patterns of English* at least partially resulted from the accommodation of such facts and insights. Thus, in some ways, it is closer to the Trubetzkoyan theory of oppositions delineated in *Grundzüge* than it is to its own base, the Jakobsonian distinctive feature theory of *Preliminaries* and *Fundamentals,* as will become apparent from this volume. Trubetzkoy's *Grundzüge,* which has been called a classic of systematization and compilation, has, of course, provided a rich source for many types of linguistic observation in current phonological theory. After an initial "Sturm und Drang" period for distinctive feature theory in generative phonology, the value of this earlier source has now also been established. A rediscovery of this source may even have been at least partially responsible for a reworking of the earlier Jakobson-based feature system.

In their inception, features in early Prague phonology were the result of the discovery of systematic regularities and correspondences between the sounds of a phonological system; they were closely related to typological studies. These regularities, subsequently characterized by the distinctive features, were thus also examined from the viewpoint of linguistic universals. Just as phonological theory expanded, shifted in emphasis, and in the course of its development made priorities out of different theoretical principles, the significance and status of the original feature concept also shifted and changed. This is particularly true of the feature concept within the context of generative theory. As noted, features in the generative framework took their roots from the Jakobsonian distinctive features. Halle, as a student and collaborator of Jakobson and as the foremost generative phonologist, appears here as the intermediary. Within the generative framework and its theoretical demands for explanatory adequacy, the relationship of the phonological component to its phonetic realization and to the rest of grammar is very complex. It is therefore not surprising that the earlier set of features can no longer fulfill all the possible requirements and theoretical priorities. In this context it is noteworthy that the ideas and concerns of Trubetzkoy and Jakobson (and their occasional disagreement) in many ways already foreshadowed what subsequently were to become leading issues in feature theory. One example is the way in which the divergent views of the two scholars foreshadowed problems related to the principle of binarity. Jakobson was the first to successfully break down the phonological system into a set of binary distinctive features. He was able to do this as early as 1938 and before his arrival in the United States. As both letters and articles attest, Trubetzkoy had been well aware of the Jakobsonian breakthrough, but in his own classificatory system he resisted following suit in the binary analysis of the point of articulation parameter. It is also noteworthy that Trubetzkoy had not as yet united vowels and consonants under one unified feature system as Jakobson later did.

It is difficult to dismiss this early difference in the approaches by the two scholars simply by an argument of a more fully versus a less fully developed feature system. Rather, it is more likely that this difference has its basis in the prioritizing of different theoretical principles, which for Jakobson included the principles of simplicity, generality, and economy. While the Jakobsonian use of a single, unified feature system for vowels and consonants at first glance seemed to adhere to these principles, it was not free from redundancies. Recent research also seems to indicate that vowels and consonants appear to correspond to different articulatory, acoustic, and perceptual parameters and realities. The Jakobsonian binary breakthough rested on a redefinition of the articulatory correlates of the point of articulation parameter for consonants. Trubetzkoy, in the development of his conceptual framework, had repeatedly stressed the importance of phonetic realism, a principle that did not necessarily seem in accord with the later Jakobsonian principle of binarity. Trubetzkoy therefore appeared to refrain consciously from following in Jakobson's footsteps. The principle of phonetic reality may also have had a lower priority for Jakobson. He was able to stretch phonetic reality ingeniously so as to redefine the articulatory correlates of the point of articulation parameter and achieve the degree of abstraction necessary for the development of a more unified feature system.

Current work in feature analysis, especially by Ladefoged and the UCLA phonetics group, also has as its goal to capture a feature system in which the phonetic ground is hugged more closely. Consequently the feature framework being developed by the Ladefoged group in many ways comes closer to a Trubetzkoyan classification then it does to the Jakobsonian classification of *Preliminaries* and *Fundamentals* (see Ladefoged, 1971).

Another point that continues to be an issue in current feature theory is the relationship between phonetics and phonology. In particular, it concerns the relationship between possible binary features on a phonological level to binary features on a phonetic level and the way such features are mapped into each other. Studies in feature analysis have shown that many of the phonological features involve the specification of more than a single phonetic parameter, a fact that had not been considered seriously enough in early investigations. It should also be pointed out that there is no reason to expect each phonological feature to be interpretable in terms of a single physical scale as is required by the current Chomsky-Halle framework. There seems to be little doubt that the Chomsky-Halle model will have to be changed to accommodate the facts uncovered in recent and ongoing articulatory, acoustic, and perceptual research (Lindau 1975; Ladefoged, 1977).

In connection with the question of the relationship between phonetics and phonology, the issue of whether the same set of features should be used on the phonological and the phonetic level also becomes relevant. This issue had not been raised in the earlier versions of distinctive feature theory, since the distinctive feature developed as a purely phonological functional concept. The inclusion of phonetics in the generative model therefore also occasioned substantial changes in the feature concept.

An additional issue in current feature theory is the type of correlate to be sought for each feature. In their inception, features tended to be described in terms of articulatory correlates. But early mentalistic and psychological influences also brought into play such notions as a speaker's linguistic consciousness and the way a sound was "felt" or perceived by a listener. A semiconcerted effort appears to have been made in the early Prague School to find acoustic or perceptual correlates for the individual features then being discovered. It is to be noted that in their early use the attributes "perceptual" and "acoustic" were used quite impressionistically and were essentially interchangeable in meaning. It appears, however, that "acoustic" was generally intended to mean "perceptual." Early feature correlates were primarily articulatory and secondarily "perceptual." The first consistent use of acoustic (in the sense of instrumentally verifiable) correlates occurred in Jakobson's *Preliminaries*. Jakobson's rationale for providing acoustic correlates rested on a perceptual basis. He wanted to come as close as possible to a hearer's point of view, although the exact perceptual correlates of the features had not been verified.

Subsequent experimental studies which have taken their incentive from these early investigations have attempted to support these earlier claims of perceptual and/or acoustic feature correlates, but they have met with only partial success (Wickelgren, 1966; Klatt, 1968; Singh, Woods, and Becker, 1972; Wang and Bilger, 1973). These studies have made it clear that the optimal choice of a feature correlate, whether articulatory, acoustic, or perceptual, very much depends on the individual feature under consideration, and that some features or feature sets are more easily characterized in terms of acoustic correlates while others are characterized more adequately in articulatory terms. There are still others that are perceptually relevant and yet have no direct articulatory or acoustic correlates. Articulatory or acoustic feature specifications may have considerable complexity, and it is possible for any one feature to have more than one simple or single articulatory and/or acoustic correlate. In addition, the choice of any particular feature system itself may also depend on the demands made on such a system. For example, the choice of articulatory or acoustic emphasis may depend on the particular use for which the feature system is intended. Once a choice has been made, there is also no simple one-to-one correspondence between one feature set and another, or between a set of articulatory and a set of acoustic or perceptual correlates within the same feature system. Feature theory thus continues to be revamped depending on what is considered important at any given moment both from a practical and a theoretical point of view.

In considering the present state of the art in feature theory, it then becomes abundantly clear that no one single set of features can fill all the demands put forth by potentially competing theoretical principles. For example, if optimal perceptual correlates have a high priority from the viewpoint of a given phonological theory, a principle espoused by Jakobson in *Preliminaries,* the optimal set of features is likely to be different from one based on the criterion of phonetic or articulatory realism. On the other hand, a feature set may take an entirely different form when its primary purpose is either to account for, in the most parsimonious way, the speech errors in spontaneous conversation and to characterize the prevalence of certain types of such error (van den Broecke and Goldstein, 1977); to account for articulatory phonetic reality and to reveal the interrelationship between phonetically related sounds (Vennemann and Ladefoged, 1973); to account for perceptual relationships and psychological space between sounds within a sound system (Singh, 1975); or to represent most economically the correspondences between a phonological and a phonetic matrix (Ladefoged, 1977). A set of features may vary further depending on whether the principle of binarity is chosen as a high ranking classificatory principle.

When viewing feature theory in its historical perspective, it is important to remember that distinctive features did not develop in isolation. They grew out of a network of related concepts and ideas. These included the concepts of markedness, natural class, morphophonemes, and neutralization. Although some of these concepts were dormant for some time, they have been rediscovered and incorporated into the generative phonological framework. Other notions have also resurfaced in the guise of new labels or labels that are only faintly reminiscent of their earlier functions, although the distinctions they signify were clearly recognized in the earlier classificatory systems. For example, the notion of first-, second-, and third-order features in the early Trubetzkoyan classification clearly reflected a hierarchical principle which was recently explored by van den Broecke (1976). Features of different rank order were also inherent in Trubetzkoy's subsequent terminological complexity in feature classification, although perhaps with a different emphasis. Vennemann and Ladefoged (1973) rediscovered this last important distinction and suggested a differentiation between "cover" features and "prime" features to capture this distinction. Some of these ideas thus already had been part of earlier considerations; they were subsequently disregarded when other classificatory or theoretical principles appeared on the scene, only to be rediscovered at a still later date.

A review of the various aspects of feature theory reveals two general areas that have always called for attention. One area is the need for empirical support for distinctive feature theory, including experimental studies and the way such studies support or falsify claims made for specific features, feature sets, or their correlates. Empirical support can also be derived from precise studies of phonological phenomena in a wide range of languages which show a particular feature or feature set to be adequate to capture the necessary phonetic detail and phonological generalizations. The second area is the need to investigate the value of feature theory vis-à-vis the types of general or specific linguistic principles which govern the popular phonological model of the moment and the selection and choice of a particular feature or set of features. Such principles include the requirement for binarity, phonetic realism, symmetry, parsimony of features or redundancy rules in a phonological component, and explanatory adequacy. This area also relates to whether language-universal or language-specific generalizations are to be emphasized.

Clearly, it would be exceedingly difficult to serve all these various purposes equally well by the same unmodified set of features. Unfortunately, it has been the case that the various requirements imposed on feature sets have not always been viewed from a holistic point of view. This often causes unwarranted and unnecessary criticism (Postal 1968; Walsch, 1974). The conceptual framework and the goals of distinctive feature theory at any one time therefore need to be clearly understood and kept in mind. Feature theory has been lauded and criticized in different ways and for various reasons. It also has been changed in various directions. To fully understand the feature concept and its application and possible variables, it becomes necessary to study its broad foundations. The present work is intended to do just that.

The book consists of two sections. The first links the feature concept to other concepts in phonology. Many of the classical ideas in phonology have experienced a rebirth within the generative framework and have been adopted into that theory in appropriately altered form and content. The origins and the development of these concepts are sketched, emphasizing their original use and meaning as compared to their status in generative theory today. The second section then outlines and discusses the foundations and developmental stages of current feature theory.

PART I
The Development of the Conceptual Framework of the Theory of Distinctive Features

De Saussure (1916) characterized phonemes as being "the first units which one obtains in segmenting the speech continuum" (p. 65) and as being "above all contrastive, relative, and negative" (p. 164). Following de Saussure, Trubetzkoy argued that any system of phonemes presupposed a system of oppositions, and any classification of phonemes presupposed a classification of oppositions. The concept of opposition was a logical one for Trubetzkoy, and it was not limited to the field of phonology. In phonology a theory of oppositions developed only gradually. Its development and that of related concepts are traced below.

A THEORY OF CORRELATIONS

In early Prague phonology, two types of phonological oppositions were considered fundamental to any phonological system: the correlations and the disjunctions. Even though no entirely uniform conception existed for the notion of correlation, this concept was to become most fruitful in the development of phonological theory.[1] In it we can already recognize the beginnings of a binary distinctive feature theory. The theory of distinctive features rests on the concept of the correlation in the sense that correlations involve the recurrence of the same phonological relationship between a series of speech sounds in a given language.

Correlations and disjunctions were seen as the two types of phonological oppositions that constituted the phonological system of a language. Correlations were those oppositions in which several contrastive pairs were differentiated by the same feature in a parallel manner. An example in English would be the series of pairs /p/-/b/, /t/-/d/, and /k/-/g/. In this example one member of the contrastive pair is unvoiced while the other is voiced. The same contrast is found in a whole series of phoneme pairs.

Disjunctions, on the other hand, were those oppositions within a phonological system in which the two members of a contrastive pair could not be distinguished by only one feature. Disjunctions involved phonemes from different correlative series that were opposed to each other by several features. An example of a disjunctive pair in English would be /d/-/p/, which are opposed to each other along the parameters of voicing and place of articulation. Elsewhere in the system each of these differentiates individually among a whole series of phoneme pairs. When acting as the sole differential characteristic between such a series, each of these features thus also forms the basis of a correlation elsewhere in the phonological system.

The notion of correlation was first introduced by Roman Jakobson in 1928, in *Proposition au Premier Congrès International de Linguistes,* co-signed by Trubetzkoy and Karcevskij. Correlation was defined as follows:

> . . . a phonological correlation consists of a series of binary oppositions which share a *common element* [principle].
> The latter can be thought of independently of each pair of opposing members. (1928/1962, p. 3; emphasis added).

In the 1931 compilation of definitions of concepts used by the Prague School, *Projet de terminologie phonologique standardisée,* this definition of correlation was followed by:

> . . . phonological system of oppositions which are characterized by a common correlational property.

All other opposition relationships which could not be subsumed under the above definition were lumped together under the term "disjunction," which in *Projet* was defined as the:

> . . . opposition of two disjunctive phonological units.[2]

The definition of correlation imposed the following two conditions on any opposition to qualify as a correlation:

1. A phonological opposition must share an element or a property (its *principe commun*) which differentiated between its two members. An example is the voicing feature in the opposition /p/-/b/ in English.
2. The same differential relationship has to be repeated in more than one phoneme pair. The voicing feature in English again may serve as an example. It is repeated in the series /p/-/b/, /t/-/d/, /k/-/g/.

The common element under condition 1 was not necessarily understood as comprising one feature only. For example, in *Polabische Studien* Trubetzkoy wrote:

> . . . those *properties* which are discriminative for each of these pairs, are abstracted by the speaker's linguistic consciousness and experienced as correlative-contrastive properties. (1929c, p. 120; emphasis added)

Subsequently, Trubetzkoy became more specific in his use of the term "common element." It later involved only one property.[3]

There was no downward limit on the number of pairs needed to fulfill condition 2 inherent in the concept of correlation. In *Die phonologischen Systeme* (1931a) Trubetzkoy specified that the relationship should extend to at least one additional pair ". . . if the same relationship is repeated in at least one other phoneme pair" (p. 97).[4]

The "common element" which in *Proposition* (Jakobson, Trubetzkoy, and Karcevskij, 1928/1962, p. 4) was also referred to as the *basis for comparison (terme de comparaison),* was replaced by *principium divisionis* in Jakobson's 1929 article, *Remarques sur l'évolution phonologique du russe comparée à celle des autres langues slaves. Principium divisionis* is roughly translatable into English as division, classificatory, or defining principle.

The classification of phonological oppositions in terms of correlations and disjunctions was an early attempt at refining phonologocal theory. However, the two concepts proved to be too vague and difficult to define and to use objectively. The distinction between them was eventually dropped. In *Proposition* and *Remarques* Jakobson discussed the concept of correlation in psychological and mentalistic terms, which seemed to reflect the influence of the Polish scholar Baudouin de Courtenay.[5] Subsequent criticism by writers such as Karl Bühler led Jakobson to re-examine the concept.[6] Jakobson had originally maintained a strict separation between correlations and disjunctions. As late as 1933, in *La phonologie actuelle,* Trubetzkoy agreed with Jakobson on this distinction. Trubetzkoy stressed the need for a better descriptive terminology, while at the same time emphasizing the importance and newness of the two concepts.[7] Jakobson considered the distinction between correlation and disjunction to be basic and essential and insisted on a strict separation between the two concepts for some time to come.[8]

Yet the distinction between correlations and disjunctions proved to be of limited theoretical value. Only a small number of phoneme relationships could be explained more fully be these two classes. The relations that were amenable to a more insightful analysis were those that were clearly in binary opposition to one another and were repeated in several phoneme pairs. Examples would include voiced versus voiceless consonants in English and nasal versus non-nasal vowels in French. Other phoneme relationships remained opaque and could not be better explained by the notion of correlation and disjunction. Examples would be the phoneme relationships characterized by place of articulation which would include oppositions between the labial, labiodental, alveolar, velar, and pharyngeal places of articulation.

The somewhat forced delimitation between correlations and disjunctions may in fact have delayed the development of phonology. The original division between the two notions broke down when finer distinctions were uncovered within the disjunctions themselves. Trubetzkoy was the first who worked out a more complex classification of oppositions. Jakobson also discarded his earlier dichotomy, but he did not replace it with any more complex classification of oppositions. Instead, he changed directly to a binary approach of oppositions. Also, he did not share in the complicated nomenclature associated with the Trubetzkoyan classification. The relationship between the Trubetzkoyan classification of oppositions and that of Jakobson is examined at a later point. Of particular interest are the similarities shared by the two systems, the aspects in which they differ, and the possible influences that each system may have had on the development of the other. However, before examining these points, related concepts need to be discussed.

PHONEME AND OPPOSITION

The Phoneme and the Opposition: Their Relation to Each Other

The relationship of the phoneme concept to the opposition concept in the early days of phonological theory is of considerable interest.

Before the Prague School developed the theory of oppositions which was to lead to a structuralist approach, phonologists held an atomistic view of the sounds of a language. In contrast to the subsequent structuralist viewpoint, the atomistic approach considered each sound to be a separate entity existing by itself without reference to its relations with the other sounds of the language. The concept of the phoneme as the smallest indivisible unit may have been a logical extension of this earlier atomistic view. As the concept of the distinctive feature ripened in the Prague School, phonemes could be seen to share elements with some but not other phonemes of a given language. Depending on the nature and number of the shared elements, subunits or distinctive features and the relationship of one phoneme to another could be formulated.

Both the notion of opposition and the notion of relativity were important concepts in the development of Prague phonology. They had originated with de Saussure, who was one of the major influences on the Prague School. As noted earlier, de Saussure viewed phonemes "as oppositive, relative, and negative entities."[9] The Prague School maintained that sounds could not be considered by themselves. Each sound had to be viewed in relation to other sounds and to the entire sound system of a given language. Partly as a result of the developing theory of oppositions, phonemes were seen to exist by virtue of their differential elements, that is, their distinctive features. This early structuralist approach stressed the coherence of language as a functioning system. Emphasis on coherence and a system approach did not only apply to phonology. It also applied to other areas of language. It was the guiding principle in the subsequent synchronic studies carried out in the structuralist movement that had developed directly out of the Prague School. In these studies language or aspects of language were viewed as a system at any point in time without reference to historic change or relatedness to other languages.

The theory of oppositions developed in conjunction with studies in phonological typology. Early Prague School interest had focused heavily on this area, which was to yield significant contributions to phonological universals. Phonological typology had also been one of Trubetzkoy's main interests. Two of his early articles, *Zur allgemeinen Theorie der phonologischen Vokalsysteme* (1929a) and *Die phonologischen Systeme* (1931a), discussed later in detail, were studies in phonological typology. At the same time these studies were also particularly relevant in tracing the conceptual development of a theory of oppositions and the structuralist point of view. Trubetzkoy is now well known as one of the major forces behind the development of Prague School structuralism.

Closely related to the structuralist point of view was the notion of phoneme content, which grew out of the concept of oppositions and their relationship to phonemes.

Notion of Phoneme Content

In examining the relationship of oppositions to phonemes, the following statements taken from Trubetzkoy's *Grundzüge der Phonologie* (1939/1969) are of interest. They date from a time when some sense of organization had already been brought into the jumble of phonological data and when phonological ideas had already begun to come to fruition. Trubetzkoy wrote in *Grundzüge:*

> ... in phonology the major role is played not by the phonemes but by the distinctive oppositions. Each phoneme has a definable phonemic content only because the system of distinctive oppositions shows a definitive order and structure. (1939/1969, p. 68)

and:

> ... the phoneme inventory of a language is naturally only a corollary of the system of distinctive oppositions. (1939/1969, p. 67)

The notion of phoneme content seems to have been a by-product of the analysis of opposition relationships. In modern terminology phoneme content may be thought of as the set of features constituting a particular phoneme. These features are distinctive; that is, they distinguish that phoneme from at least one other phoneme in the same system. Trubetzkoy defined phoneme content in his culminating work *Grundzüge* as "the sum of the phonologically relevant properties of a phoneme" (1939/1969, p. 36).

The notion of phoneme content appears rather early in phonological development. Trubetzkoy explicitly called attention to it in his *Zur allgemeinen Theorie der phonologischen Vokalsysteme* (1929a). There he referred to it in mentalistic terms as "psychological content," distinguishing between "features" *(Merkmale)* and "image elements" *(Vorstellungselemente).* He considered features phonetic in character while he considered image elements phonological in nature. Trubetzkoy maintained that only the image elements were important for the psychological content of the phonemes. The following example illustrates the difference. Given a "k" sound in German and Kyak-Cherkess (a Caucasian language), Trubetzkoy argued that although all motor-acoustic features for this sound were identical in German and Kyak-Cherkess, only two features of "k" were also image elements, that is, distinctive, for German, while six features were image elements for Kyak-Cherkess. The psychological content of the "k" in German therefore consisted of two image elements. Hence it was "simple." The psychological content of the "k" in Kyak-Cherkess consisted of six image elements. Hence it was "complex."

The reason for this quantitative difference in psychological content hinged on the fact that psychological content was determined by the entire phonological system. The distinction between simple and complex content was due to the fact that psychological content was determined within the framework of correlations and disjunctions. Within this framework it was only possible to analyze those phonemes whose motor-acoustic features also recurred in other phonemes of the same system, that is, were correlative. As noted earlier, correlations were oppositions that differentiated among members of a series of phoneme pairs by a common element. Disjunctions were all other types of oppositions in which a common element did not differentiate between more than one phoneme pair. Phoneme relationships were analyzable only insofar as they were also correlative. Disjunctive phoneme relationships were initially unanalyzable. Phoneme content was complex or simple depending on the ratio of correlative and disjunctive oppositions in a system. The greater the ratio of correlations to disjunctions in a given system, the greater the complexity of the content of each phoneme in that system. The greater the ratio of disjunctions to correlations in a given system, the greater the opacity of that system and the simpler the content of each phoneme, hence the difference between German and Kyak-Cherkess in terms of phoneme content. Also, the more phonemes a language had, the more features could potentially also occur. A higher number of such features could then also be potentially correlative and provide for "image elements."

The following example represents differences in phoneme content of the /k/ in German and Kyak-Cherkess, (after *Zur allgemeinen Theorie der phonologischen Vokalsysteme*, 1929a/ 1964, p. 109):

Phoneme content in terms of image elements for /k/ in German:

1. Tenuis
2. Dorsal occlusive

Phoneme content in terms of image elements for /k/ in Kyak-Cherkess:

1. Voicelessness
2. Lenis (opposed to geminate k)
3. Infraglottal expiration (as opposed to glottalized k)
4. Unroundedness (as opposed to rounded k)
5. Prevelarity (as opposed to postvelar k)
6. Dorsality (as opposed to apicality)

As the above example shows, the distinction between correlations and disjunctions contributed to the opacity of phoneme content in the early stages of feature development. The situation was remedied when finer distinctions were uncovered within the disjunctions themselves and the earlier distinction between the two notions was dropped.

The mentalistic terminology which had been associated with phoneme content in its early beginnings also soon disappeared. Psychological content subsequently simply became phoneme content, as illustrated by Trubetzkoy's 1935 article, *Anleitung zu phonologischen Beschreibungen*. The distinction between the earlier "features" *(Merkmale)* and "image elements" *(Vorstellungselemente)* was also dropped. In *Anleitung*, Trubetzkoy already stressed the need for phonological descriptions to account for phonemic content and to specify such content as an aspect of the description. As noted earlier, the notion of phoneme content was defined in *Grundzüge* "as the sum of the phonologically relevant properties of a phoneme" (1939/1969, p. 36). It is essentially in this sense that it was taken over into modern phonology.

Development of the Phoneme Concept:
Its Relation to the Feature Concept

Many attempts at a clear definition of the phoneme were made throughout the development of the Prague School. An early definition of the phoneme in *Projet de terminologie phonologique standardisée* (1931) had been: " . . . [a] phonological unit which cannot be analyzed into smaller and simpler phonological units."[10] A phoneme definition in this form was obviously insufficient in the light of further developments and ultimately could not survive. It was inconsistent with the subsequently developed definition of phoneme content as "the sum of the phonologically relevant properties of a phoneme" (Trubetzkoy 1939/1969) and with the notion of the divisibility of the phoneme into still smaller elements. It is clear from what has been said earlier that the phoneme definition given in *Projet* was not the definition which Trubetzkoy followed in practice. It also was not the first definition by which the Prague School operated.

In the earliest days, both Trubetzkoy and Jakobson, under the influence of Baudouin de Courtenay, had spoken of phonemes as "sound images" *(Lautvorstellungen)*. Thus, in *Thèses presentées au premier congrès des philologues slaves* (1929) in line with this conceptualization phonemes were considered as "the simplest, meaning-differentiating acoustic-motor images in a given language."[11] The "meaning-differentiating . . . images" referred to the distinctive function of the phoneme, which has always been an integral part of the phoneme concept in the Prague School. It reflected the influence of Ščerba and the Russian School. Ščerba had defined the phoneme as:

> . . . the shortest generic phonetic representation possible for a given language, which can be associated with semantic representations and which can serve to differentiate words.[12]

The mentalistic conceptualization of the phoneme reflected in the use of the term "image" was subsequently also abandoned. In *Grundzüge* Trubetzkoy called the concept of the sound image *(Lautvorstellung)* a mistake, because, he said:

> . . . acoustic-motor images correspond to every phonetic variant inasmuch as the articulation is regulated and controlled by the speaker . . . there is no reason to consider some of these images as conscious and others as subconscious. (1939/1969, p. 38)

However, a better operational definition of the phoneme concept, which would be in harmony with the development of the theory of oppositions, was still to be finalized. After Trubetzkoy abandoned the term "sound image" he replaced it with the term "sound intent" *(Lautabsicht)*, which was yet another quasi-mentalistic conceptualization.

In his paper to the Second International Congress of Linguists in Geneva in 1931, Trubetzkoy noted:

> Phonology is not concerned with sounds as physical phenomena, but with phonemes, that is to say, with *sound intents* living in the linguistic consciousness and realized in speech sounds. . . . Only those sound differences which, in a given language, can be used to differentiate meaning, have phonological validity, for only those are *intentional* from the point of view of the particular linguistic system. . . . The phonological system of a language is the sum total of the sound *intents* which perform a meaning-differentiating function in a given language. (Trubetzkoy, 1933b, p. 109; emphasis added)

This definition, too, was still couched in mentalistic terms. It was subsequently abandoned by Trubetzkoy because, as he explained in *Grundzüge*:

> . . . the expression "sound intent" . . . was actually only an alternative phrasing of the designation of the phoneme as sound image. Consequently it was also wrong. (1939/1969, p. 38)

It is noteworthy that Trubetzkoy's paper to the Second International Congress of Linguists also included a more general reference to the phoneme. In alternating the terms "sound intent" *(Lautabsicht)* and "sound concept" *(Lautbegriff)*, Trubetzkoy explained:

> A sound always contains an entire complex of phonetic features. The phonetician must examine all these features. However, *to differentiate meaning, only a few features of a particular sound need to be examined, the remainder being irrelevant for this purpose.* Phonology is interested *only in "sound concepts" abstracted from all features irrelevant for the distinction of meaning.* (Trubetzkoy, 1933b, p. 121; emphasis added)

This statement, together with the discussion of phoneme content in Trubetzkoy's *Zur allgemeinen Theorie* (1929a), already clearly encompassed the concept of the phoneme as a bundle of distinctive features. Jakobson subsequently proposed just such a definition. It was first published in 1932 in a Czech encyclopedia (see Jakobson, 1932b). Its original formulation in translation, as it appears in *Selected Writings I,* is as follows:

> . . . the phoneme . . . by this term we designate a set of those concurrent sound properties which are used in a given language to distinguish words of unlike meaning. (Jakobson, 1962c, p. 231)

This is essentially also the definition which Trubetzkoy adopted for *Grundzüge*:

> . . . one can say that the phoneme is the sum of the phonologically relevant properties of a sound. (1939/1969, p. 36)

Trubetzkoy coupled this definition with yet another one:

> Those phonological units which, from the point of view of the given language, cannot be analyzed into still smaller successive units, are called phonemes. (1939/1969, p. 35)

Trubetzkoy's above definitions were, of course, quite compatible with each other. The former referred to what can be called the paradigmatic axis of the phoneme and what had previously been considered phoneme content. The latter referred to the syntagmatic axis of the phoneme and its occurrence in a chain of sounds.

The conception of the phoneme as a bundle of distinctive features was the direct result of the analysis of oppositive relationships. More specifically, it was a consequence of the study of phoneme content. The analysis of phonemic content in turn was facilitated and could be carried out with greater clarity after the original distinction between correlations and disjunctions had been discarded as insufficient and replaced by a new classification. (This is discussed later, on p. 51 ff.) As already pointed out, within the earlier framework of correlations and disjunctions the notion of phoneme content had remained largely opaque. In earlier definitions of the phoneme, phoneme content had not come into play at all.

Thus, the first definition of the phoneme as a bundle of distinctive features actually dates from 1932. It seems improbable that the full extent of its implications was recognized at the time. It also seems clear that the conception of the phoneme as a bundle of distinctive features can already be inferred from Trubetzkoy's work predating 1932. It is a curious fact, however, that even though Trubetzkoy appeared to have been operating with the above conception of the phoneme as a composite unit, he nevertheless paid lip service to the definition as it appeared in *Projet*. He did so, surprisingly, as late as 1936, as is evident from his work, *Essai d'une théorie des oppositions phonologiques*.[13] It deserves to be pointed out, however, that at the time he wrote this essay he did not attach much importance to definitions. He was more concerned with practical work.[14]

Another point becomes extremely important in the development of feature theory and the relationship between the phoneme and the distinctive feature. Originally, the phoneme had been considered a member of an opposition. This later changed, and the distinctive feature itself ultimately became the member of an opposition. To follow the course of this shift, yet another Praguian definition of the phoneme must be highlighted. This definition emphasized the phoneme as a member of an opposition. In *Remarques sur l'évolution phonologique du russe comparée à celle des autres langues slaves* Jakobson defined the phoneme as:

> . . . that repertory of oppositions which in a given language can be associated with differentiating meanings. *All members of a phonological opposition which cannot be broken down* into smaller phonological sub-oppositions *are called phonemes*. (1929/1962, p. 10; emphasis added)[15]

In other words, phonemes were here defined as being the smallest unanalyzable units in the phonological system. When the phoneme was redefined as a bundle of distinctive features, a further shift in the meanings of phoneme, opposition, and distinctive feature took place.

Originally, then, phonemes were thought to be the basic units of oppositions. However, based on the fact that no phoneme could have a "single, predictable opposite" Jakobson subsequently transferred the oppositive value from the phoneme to the distinctive feature. This, according to Jakobson himself, was done in *Zur Struktur des Phonems* (1939), where he reasoned as follows:

> . . . the oppositions of distinctive properties are real, logical, binary oppositions. By definition, either member of such an opposition includes the opposing member. In contrast, the relationship between two phonemes is complex and can consist of several oppositions. By definition the number of phonemic distinctions is higher than the number of phonemes. . . . In contrast, the number of distinctive properties or their oppositions is considerably smaller. (1939c/1962, p. 303)

> The phoneme is a complex unit which can be completely analyzed into distinctive properties. These purely contrastive properties cannot be broken down any further, and constitute the constant, basic units of a phonological system. (1939c/1962, p. 310)

The stage was now set for a consistent development of distinctive features as we know them from *Preliminaries to Speech Analysis* (1952) and *Fundamentals of Language* (1956).

In summary, it is evident that the concept of distinctive features did not develop all at once. Several steps can be identified in its development, and several related notions were significant and need to be taken into consideration. The first step in the unfolding of the concept was the distinction between correlations and disjunctions. Even though this distinction had to be ultimately abandoned, it was significant in early development. Associated with it was the recognition of the existence of different types of contrastive relationships within a phonological system. The concept of phoneme content followed this discovery of oppositive relationships. The exploration of phoneme content in turn ultimately led to the definition of the phoneme as a bundle of distinctive features. Even though earlier definitions of the phoneme within Prague School phonology had included considerations of the entire system and had incorporated the notions of relativity and opposition, the development of the distinctive feature concept would not have been possible without such an exploration.

These developments, in turn, subsequently required a shift of the notion of opposition from the phoneme to the feature level. It is clear that the concept of distinctive feature could not have developed in the context of an atomistic view of the sounds of a language. Inherent in the development of the distinctive feature was the Praguian recognition that there was coherence between the sounds of a language as a system and that the value of each sound depended on its relationship with the other sounds of that system. Hence, the value of each sound or phoneme was relative. The reality of the phoneme came first, and then that of the distinctive feature, which depended on the structure of a given phonemic system. In this sense, both were abstract constructs.

The recognition that phonemes constituted further divisible units can be viewed as a factor in the abandonment of the earlier mentalistic framework, since it seemed to make their study more concrete. A shift away from mentalism can also be viewed as reflecting the general trends of the times, which showed their influence in other sciences, for example, in psychology, where the earlier mentalistic approaches were replaced by a new model, that of behaviorism.

So far, distinctive features have not necessarily been discussed in binary terms. How distinctive features gradually developed into a binary system is discussed later on, as are the respective roles of Trubetzkoy and Jakobson in the development of a binary classification. Of concern here is how the final Praguian concept of the phoneme and the distinctive feature ultimately fared in generative phonology in terms of intrinsic content.

Even though distinctive feature theory as it is currently used in generative phonology can clearly be traced to its Praguian roots, several changes took place. First of all, generative phonologists do not operate with phonemes but with morphophonemes. In *The Sound Pattern of English* Chomsky and Halle defined the distinctive feature as:

> . . . minimal elements of which phonetic, lexical, and phonological transcriptions are composed, by combination and concatenation. (1968, p. 6).

This conception of the distinctive feature is clearly not equivalent to the distinctive feature as found in Jakobson's original phoneme definition. In *Phoneme and phonology* the phoneme had been defined as:

> . . . a set of those concurrent sound properties which are used in a given language to distinguish words of unlike meaning. (1932b/ 1962, p. 231)

Nor is this definition equivalent to the "phonologically relevant" or "distinctive properties" of Trubetzkoy's *Grundzüge*. These two older definitions refer to meaning-differentiating properties only. In contrast, the distinctive feature concept as used by Chomsky and Halle makes no distinction between phonologically relevant and phonologically irrelevant features. The distinctive feature concept thus appears to have undergone a change in meaning. It now simply stands for feature, "distinctive" having lost its specific meaning.[16]

Chomsky and Halle made a basic distinction between classificatory and phonetic functions of their distinctive features. Only in their classificatory function are distinctive features strictly binary. In their phonetic function distinctive features appear as nonbinary and receive a physical interpretation.[17] The way in which the conversion from one matrix to the other—from the classificatory to the phonetic, or vice versa—is to be carried out, still awaits definitive exploration and remains outside this discussion. However, Chomsky and Halle did stipulate that this conversion take place in the phonological component of their framework.

An additional concept important in *The Sound Pattern of English* was a newly introduced concept, that of the *alphabetic symbol*. In accordance with descriptivist practice, the notation for the alphabetic symbol is written between two slashes to signify phonemic status. Chomsky and Halle defined these alphabetic symbols "with their conventional interpretation as abbreviation for feature sets" loosely as:

> . . . nothing more than convenient ad hoc abbreviations for feature bundles introduced for ease of printing and reading but without *systematic import*. (1968, p. 64; emphasis added)

It thus seems that the original relationship between the distinctive feature and the phoneme was lost. Additionally, features in the Chomsky-Halle framework were not necessarily distinctive anymore. As noted, Trubetzkoy had defined the phoneme as "the sum of phonologically relevant properties of a sound" (1939/ 1969, p. 36).

The Chomsky and Halle term, *"systematic import,"* must be taken as intrinsic to the definition itself. Based on their definition of *"alphabetic symbol"* and ignoring the use of the notational slashes, the Chomsky-Halle alphabetic symbol seems to resemble more closely the earlier conception of the speech sound, which Trubetzkoy had defined as follows:

> . . . speech sounds . . . are the sum of all distinctive as well as non-distinctive phonic properties occurring at a specific point in the sound flow. (1939/1969, p. 37)

Also, Chomsky and Halle referred to their alphabetic symbol as a *"feature set"* or *"feature complex"* (p. 64), a term that they further subdefined. A feature complex (or set) was a *unit* if it is fully specified, and an *archi-unit* if it is not fully specified.

The archi-unit cannot be considered equivalent to the earlier phoneme concept, which included *all the distinctive features, but only those features which were distinctive* (Jakobson, 1932; Trubetzkoy 1939/1969). In the earlier interrelationship between phoneme and distinctive features, only the phonologically irrelevant properties were not specified. Once the features for a particular phoneme had been determined, this feature specification never varied. In contrast, the specification of features in the Chomsky-Halle archi-unit could vary since context was a factor to be considered in the specification of the archi-unit. Thus the features indicated for an archi-unit could differ as a result of the place of the archi-unit in a sound sequence. One and the same alphabetic symbol could therefore have several archi-units depending on which features were specified.

Chomsky and Halle divided their feature complex or unit even further. If a unit contained the feature *segment,* it was called *segment.* If it did not contain the feature *segment,* that is, if it contained the feature −*segment,* it was called *boundary.* An *archi-segment,* then, was an archi-unit that also contained the feature +*segment.*

This additional categorization points up a further distinction with respect to the original meaning of the feature concept. Its meaning here had been expanded so as to include + and − *segment,* which in actual fact was no feature at all but only referred to a feature slot. A similar comment can also be made for other features introduced into the Chomsky-Halle feature framework, such as + and − *foreign.* Although this type of feature is also considered binary, it somehow has a different intrinsic content from the original feature definition. Furthermore, it does not seem possible to convert this type of feature into any kind of n-ary phonetic matrix. Instead, an either-or principle seems to apply.

On the other hand, an important parallel can be established in another area when comparing the current feature framework with that of the Prague School. As noted, Trubetzkoy claimed quite early that distinctive features were "image elements." He ascribed psychological reality to his distinctive features. Subsequently, the Prague School tried to rid its definitions of mentalism and psychologism. Chomsky and Halle would also claim that their features have psychological content and that they are phonetically real to the speaker. But while in the earlier Prague School, psychological reality was ascribed only to the distinctive features, in expanding the use of the feature concept Chomsky and Halle also expanded the range of application of psychological reality. The question of psychological reality and its corollaries is discussed in more detail later (see p. 158 ff.).

Summarizing then, when the concept of the original distinctive feature is compared to its subsequent conceptualization in generative phonology, several radical changes can be observed:

1. The distinctive feature has been completely divorced from the framework of the phoneme. It now exists as an independent entity, the phoneme having lost its place in the generative framework.

2. The meaning of distinctiveness also appears to have been lost. Distinctive features are no longer "distinctive" in their original sense and now simply stand for feature.

3. The meaning of feature has been expanded to include such distinctions as +/− segment and +/− foreign. Such distinctions are not on the same level as the original feature distinctions.

4. Changes also occurred in number and type of the originally established features. (These are discussed later in their appropriate place in this text.)

5. The concept of binarity, the development of which is discussed below, was retained only for the classificatory features. Binary features in the classificatory matrix are converted to a scale with n-ary points representing these features in a phonetic matrix. For example, the Chomsky-Halle classificatory feature +/− *front* in the phonetic matrix may represent points along a continuum. This is different from the distinction between phonologically relevant and irrelevant features, since within that framework irrelevant or nondistinctive features are still mainly binary. The distinction between classificatory and phonetic features, however, did not

resolve what Chomsky and Halle referred to as the "fruitless debate" on the binary aspect of the Jakobsonian features (cf. note 17), a debate that had been strictly on a phonological level. It included specific phonological distinctions and had little to do with any specific n-ary phonetic scale. Chomsky and Halle had claimed that the failure to distinguish clearly between abstract phonological features and concrete phonetic features had been one of the main causes for continued arguments about the binary character of the Jakobsonian distinctive features.

THE CONCEPTS OF ARCHIPHONEME, MORPHOPHONEME, MARKEDNESS, AND NEUTRALIZATION IN PRAGUE PHONOLOGY: THEIR EVOLUTION AND TREATMENT IN THE GENERATIVE FRAMEWORK

The concepts of the archiphoneme, morphophoneme, markedness, and neutralization were discoveries in the Prague School that had far reaching consequences in the subsequent development of phonological theory. They also greatly influenced generative phonology. As with the distinctive feature concept, these other four concepts underwent a considerable evolution, and the changes that occurred will be readily apparent in the coming discussion.

The concepts of the archiphoneme, morphophoneme, markedness, and neutralization did not exist in total clarity from the time of their conception. In fact, it can be claimed that confusion existed from the very start, and considerable divergence in thought became apparent in their definition and the range of their application. As these concepts received practical application in the study of a wide variety of languages, several problem areas relating to their use could be identified. A comparison of the way these notions are now used in generative phonology with the way they were conceived earlier is revealing. A statement taken from Halle's "Phonology in Generative Grammar" (1962) serves as a useful starting point. In that exposition Halle wrote:

> We may note that the idea of representing segments in a given form by less than their normal complement of features is essentially identical with the "archiphoneme" concept that was first proposed by Jakobson in *Travaux du Cercle linguistique de Prague II* (1928) and was used for a time by the Prague school. Since the Prague school did not operate consistently with features but rather regarded the phoneme as the ultimate phonological entity, great dif-

ficulties were soon experienced with this concept, which ultimately led to its official abandonment. (p. 341)

This statement had been made with respect to the representation of phonological segments in not fully specified form. It invites several comments. First, it is not too far from the truth to call the "not completely specified feature segment" or archi-unit of generative phonology essentially identical with the Praguian archiphoneme concept, even though the archiphoneme concept has been considerably expanded in the Halle conception, as seen below. It is not quite correct to maintain that the phoneme was considered the ultimate phonological entity in Prague phonology. It would, of course, depend, on whether "ultimate" refers to an analysis downward or upward. Although the Prague School did not consistently operate in terms of features, the phoneme had been defined by Jakobson as early as 1932 as "the sum of phonologically relevant properties of a sound." When Halle speaks of "official abandonment" of the concept, his statement also deserves some modification and clarification.

Changes in the Concept of Archiphoneme

The term "archiphoneme" was first proposed by Roman Jakobson. Although Jakobson abandoned the concept in his later writings, Trubetzkoy never did. In his *Retrospect* (1962b), Jakobson also appears to show a desire to re-enlist its usefulness. (In this context, also see Ivić, 1965, p. 43.)

Jakobson had coined the term "archiphoneme" in his 1929 *Remarques sur l'évolution phonologique du russe*. However, the earlier programmatic *Proposition au Premier Congrès International de Linguistes* (1928) had already implied such a unit in the context of the definition of phonological correlation:

> A phonological correlation consists of a series of binary oppositions which share a common defining element. Such an element can be thought of independent of each contrastive pair... (Jakobson, Karcevskij, and Trubetzkoy, 1928/1962, p. 3)

In *Remarques* the concept was made explicit and given a name:

> ... on the other hand, one can, of course, also abstract the common element which unite the two members of an opposition, and this substratum constitutes a kind of realistic unit in the phonological system. (1929/1962, p. 19)

And:

> . . . we can isolate a new basic entity for phonology, that of the
> *archiphoneme*. On the one hand, the archiphoneme should not be
> analyzable into smaller disjunctive phonemic oppositions. On the
> other, it should also not have a common substratum with another
> archiphoneme which can be isolated through one's linguistic con-
> sciousness. (1929/1962, p. 12; emphasis added)

Jakobson went on to specify that:

> . . . the archiphoneme should not form a correlation with another
> archiphoneme. The archiphoneme is a generic concept, it is an
> abstract unit which can unite one or several pairs of correlative
> variants (correlative phonemes). (1929/1962, p. 12)

Thus, the archiphoneme concept had originally depended on the
concept of correlation (see p. 3 ff.). Only those phoneme pairs
which formed members of a correlation or which were differentiated by the presence or the absence of a property could have an
archiphoneme.

Originally, the idea of the archiphoneme comprised both the
common core of a phoneme pair which was not differentiated by
more than one property, and the common core of more than one
phoneme pair. In the second case, each phoneme pair was differentiated by one property from the next phoneme pair. In *Retrospect* (1962b, p. 635) Jakobson only made reference to the archiphoneme in its more limited sense, as "the common core of two
phonemes within a correlative pair."

The archiphoneme concept was taken over by Trubetzkoy,
who subsequently combined it was the concept of neutralization
and made it famous. In Trubetzkoy's writings the first reference
to the archiphoneme occurs in *Polabische Studien,* where he relates it to his own, somewhat picturesque expression "phoneme
nests" *(Phonemennester):*

> . . . such a *phoneme nest* is always based on a rather blurred sound
> image, which is free from all correlative properties. Roman Jakob-
> son suggests the expression "archiphoneme" to refer to it. (1929c,
> p. 133)

The sound image—free from all correlative properties—is thus
the archiphoneme.

When the archiphoneme is defined in the 1931 *Projet de terminologie phonologique standardisée,* its meaning appears less
restricted:

> . . . [the archiphoneme] can be conceived of as the common core of
> two or several correlative phonemes after the correlative properties
> have been abstracted.

Although Jakobson's definition of the archiphoneme specified that *"the archiphoneme should not form a correlation with any other archiphoneme,"* the above definition only says that the archiphoneme can be "conceived of as . . . ," thus appearing less restrictive.

The *Projet* lists the following among examples from Russian to illustrate the archiphoneme concept:

> . . . archiphoneme . . . t after abstraction of its palatalized and unpalatalized feature (t/t'), the hard apical occlusive, after abstraction of its voiced or voiceless feature (d/t), or else, the apical occlusive, after abstraction of its palatalized, unpalatalized, voiced, and voiceless features.

$$t \, / \, t'$$

$$d \, / \, d'$$

A comparison of the definition of the archiphoneme as it is given in *Projet* with that in Jakobson's *Remarques sur l'évolution phonologique du russe* reveals two important changes. The first is that the mentalistic terminology used in *Remarques* was abandoned in *Projet*. The second is that the archiphoneme concept of *Remarques* seems more restricted than the definition given in the subsequent *Projet*. In *Projet* the common core of /t-t'/ and /d-d'/ was considered as one archiphoneme, but the common core of each pair by itself could also be considered an archiphoneme. In *Remarques* the relationship between /t-t'/ and /d-d'/ would have to be considered as that of two archiphonemes in a correlative relationship to each other. In accordance with the definition given there, though, this would have been undesirable. Therefore, there was only one choice in the case of Russian, namely, having one archiphoneme for all four phonemes.

In addition to the notion of archiphoneme, Jakobson also introduced the concept of the "fundamental variant of an archiphoneme" *(variante fondamentale d'un archiphonème),* which he defined as follows:

> . . . the fundamental variant of a phoneme or (archiphoneme respectively) is that combinatory extragrammatical (or correlative) phoneme or archiphoneme which is least dependent on contextual conditions, and which in terms of frequency, occurs in the largest and least complicated number of distinctive positions in a language. The variant which is least dependent on contextual conditions is the one which is found in the most varied environments. (1929/1962, p. 15)

In this definition, the fundamental variant of a phoneme and the fundamental variant of an archiphoneme are subject to the same conditions. In *Projet,* on the other hand, a separate definition is given for "fundamental or basic archiphoneme" *(archiphoneme fondamentale).* This definition seems to do away with the restrictions on the original definition of the archiphoneme in Jakobson's *Remarques sur l'évolution phonologique du russe.* The fundamental archiphoneme in *Projet* is defined as:

> . . . a phonological unit which, on the one hand, should not form a correlation with another phonological unit, and on the other hand should not be analyzable into smaller disjunctions. Therefore, the basic archiphonemes of a given language are constituted by those archiphonemes from which all correlational properties have been abstracted, and by unpaired phonemes, after all correlations of that language have been accounted for.

Some of the basic archiphonemes of Russian, illustrative of the above definition, and given in *Projet* cover:

$$t / t' \quad s / s' \quad s \quad r / r'$$
$$d / d' \quad z / z' \quad z$$

Trubetzkoy Adds Neutralization to the Archiphoneme Concept

Trubetzkoy had combined the Jakobsonian concept of archiphoneme with his own concept of neutralization. The first detailed exposition of neutralization is found in *Aufhebung der phonologischen Gegensätze* (1936b). Although Trubetzkoy had not used the term "neutralization" in the earlier *Polabische Studien* (1929), the development of the concept was clearly foreshadowed:

> Thus a phoneme is not always conceived of with equal clarity. While in some environments all properties of a phoneme emerge distinctly in one's linguistic consciousness, in others some properties of the same phoneme *pale* and are perceived quite indistinctly. (1929c, p. 125ff.; emphasis added)

Trubetzkoy used the concept of neutralization in an incidental manner in *Die Konsonantensysteme der østkaukasischen Sprachen* (1931e) and for some time thereafter. Subsequently, in his *Charakter und Methode der systematischen phonologischen Darstellung einer gegebenen Sprache* (1933c), the concept of neutralization had already evolved somewhat further. There Trubetzkoy discussed three types of limitations in the occurrence of phonemes. These limitations depended on whether phoneme sequences, isolated phonemes, or phonological oppositions were involved. When a sequence of phonemes could not occur in a given environment or when the phonological pattern of a language did not permit its occurrence, such limitations did not affect the total number of phonemes in a given language nor did they affect the content of individual phonemes. Their sole consequence was a limitation of the total number of permissible phoneme sequences in a given language. If a specific phoneme could not occur in a given position, such as an initial /s/ in German, the number of possible phoneme combinations was limited and the total number of phonemes which could occur in a given position was reduced. However, the phoneme content was left unchanged. In contrast, the third type of limitation of a phoneme in a particular environment involved the neutralization of a phonological opposition. In such cases not only were the number of possible phonemes in a particular environment reduced and the number of possible phoneme sequences limited, but the content of the phonemes in the position of neutralization was also changed. Trubetzkoy therefore considered neutralization of phonological properties the most important of all restrictions on occurrence.

Trubetzkoy was well aware of the implications of his theories. He warned against confusing the element which occurred in the position of neutralization with the unmarked phoneme. According to him there was a basic difference between the simple absence of a property and the active negation of that phonological property. He maintained that the neutralized phoneme existed as a unit which was independent of the phoneme pair of the neutralized opposition, in the linguistic consciousness of the speaker and the hearer.

Although in his 1933 *Character und Methode* Trubetzkoy had claimed that most cases of neutralization only involved correlative pairs, he conceded that neutralization did not entirely preclude disjunctive oppositions. It could also include more than two phonemes. Trubetzkoy illustrated this last point by the case of nasals in Sanskrit. Sanskrit has a special nasal symbol *(anusvara)* for the neutralized nasal. However, cases involving the neutralization of more than one phoneme pair or involving disjunctive oppositions were not mentioned in *Aufhebung der phonologischen Gegensätze* (1936b) or in his culminating work, *Grundzüge der Phonologie* (1939/1969) (but see below, p. 26 ff).

Subsequently, in his full blown theory of oppositions as it appears in *Grundzüge,* Trubetzkoy made a basic distinction between those oppositions which could be neutralized and those which could not (see discussion 1939/1969, p.78). His neutralizable oppositions formed a subcategory in his bilateral/multilateral dichotomy, discussed further below (also see Figure 1, p. 53).

The distinction between bilateral and multilateral oppositions was an important one in the context of the archiphoneme and neutralization. Bilateral oppositions were those in which the sum of shared features was only common to one phoneme pair. They did not recur in their totality in any other phoneme pair of the same system. An example of such a bilateral opposition would be the German phoneme pair /d/-/t/. The sum of features shared by these two phonemes is unique to that opposition and does not recur in its totality in any other phoneme pair.

Oppositions were considered multilateral when the sum of shared features also recurred in one or several other phonemes of the same system. An illustration of a multilateral opposition would be the phoneme pair /p/-/t/ in German since their common features are also shared by /k/.

Bilateral oppositions were oppositions that could be neutralized and share an underlying archiphoneme, for example, /d/-/t/ in German. The /d/ is neutralized in the syllable-final position, as in the singular and plural forms of the noun *Bund* (/bʊnt/), *Bünde* (/bʊndə/) ("bundle, bundles").

Trubetzkoy made the following comments regarding neutralization and bilateral oppositions in *Die Aufhebung der phonologischen Gegensätze:*

> In those positions where a neutralizable opposition is in effect neutralized, the specific features of an opposition member lose their phonological relevance. Only those features shared by both opposition members remain relevant. One of the members of the opposition in question thus becomes the representative of the "archiphoneme" in the position of neutralization. [Trubetzkoy then emphasized that the archiphoneme was to be understood as "the sum of all features shared by the two phonemes."] . . . only *bilateral oppositions can be neutralized.* (1936b/1964, p. 189; emphasis added)

By making the concept of the archiphoneme dependent on the concept of neutralization, Trubetzkoy restricted the domain of its application: archiphonemes were recognized only where neutralization took place. Neutralization, in turn, only took place in bilateral oppositions. Since bilateral oppositions in essence were distinguished by a single feature, the difference between two phonemes which had a common underlying archiphoneme could not consist of more than one feature either. This delimitation in the meaning of the term had not been true of its earlier application. The two opposition members of a neutralizable contrast in this limited sense could thus be equated as archiphoneme plus zero and archiphoneme plus a specific feature, respectively.

Following his definition in *Aufhebung*, Trubetzkoy clarified the concept of the archiphoneme in *Grundzüge:*

> By the term "archiphoneme" we understand the sum of distinctive features that two phonemes have in common. (1939/1969, p. 79)

and:

> ... only bilateral oppositions can be neutralized. In effect, only those oppositions that can be contrasted with all other phonological units of a given system have archiphonemes. (1939/1969, p.79)

Based on the above formulations, the archiphoneme concept should have been limited to no more than two phonemes. The same applies to the concept of neutralization. However, in *Grundzüge* is an extension of the latter concept in essentially two directions; one relates to the concept of correlations, which had been newly defined in *Grundzüge* (1939/1969, p. 83 ff.), the other to the notion of multilateral oppositions (1939/1969, p. 168).

The *Grundzüge* concept of the archiphoneme holds that only two phonemes can be involved. A correlation was defined there as "the sum of all correlation pairs characterized by the same correlation mark" (p. 85) and a correlation pair as "two phonemes that are in a relation of logically privative, proportional, bilateral opposition with each other" (cf. below, p. 66 ff.).

Privative oppositions occurred when one member of the phoneme pair exhibited the presence of a certain feature while the other member exhibited its absence. For example, in the English phoneme pair /t/-/d/, the /t/ is unvoiced and the /d/ is voiced. Correlations could form correlation bundles which were linked to one another by one common feature. For example, Sanskrit has the following correlation bundles:

$$p / p^h \quad k / k^h \quad t / t^h$$

$$b / b^h \quad g / g^h \quad d / d^h \qquad \qquad \text{etc.}$$

Correlation bundles could vary in size in terms of number of phonemes involved. Even though Trubetzkoy continued to restrict neutralization to bilateral oppositions, he maintained that entire correlation bundles could be neutralized, resulting in one underlying archiphoneme. The archiphoneme which resulted from neutralizing entire correlation bundles was not in keeping with Trubetzkoy's earlier definition of the term. As will be recalled, Trubetzkoy's archiphoneme could only involve two phonemes. However, it came close to the original archiphoneme concept of Jakobson's earlier *Remarques sur l'evolution phonologique du russe.*

Trubetzkoy's second extension of the archiphoneme concept can be found in his discussions of several languages, where he permitted multilateral oppositions to become involved in the concept of the archiphoneme. Here, he allowed neutralization in multilateral oppositions despite his previous restrictions. Without referring to the above definitions, Trubetzkoy cited the behavior of the nasals in Tamil (m,ṇ,ŋ, and ṇ) are in the central Chinese dialects (m,n,ŋ, and ɲ) as instances of neutralization. In Tamil, nasals assimilate to the following obstruents. In the central Chinese dialects only n and ɲ are found finally, ŋ after back vowels and n after front vowels.

Trubetzkoy's earlier restrictions on the definitions of the archiphoneme and neutralization notwithstanding we read in *Grundzüge* with respect to the above examples:

> All these cases thus involve the neutralization of multilateral oppositions between all nasals, and only in this way is neutralization possible, that is, viewed only in this fashion is it possible to speak of a resultant archiphoneme that can be distinguished by specific phonological properties from all other phonemes that occur in that position. . . . the specific properties of the "indeterminate" nasal (or of the nasal archiphoneme) are its nasal resonance and its sonorant character, i.e., its minimal degree of obstruction. (1939/1969, p. 168)

Even though several phonemes were involved in a multilateral opposition relationship, only one feature per phoneme was neutralized. Trubetzkoy termed that feature the "specific localization property *(Lokalisierungeigenschaft)*" of that phoneme.

Trubetzkoy had clearly pointed out that a phonological description also needed to account for the absence of certain phonemes in particular environments (1939/1969, p. 242). These could also have been considered instances of neutralization. However, where such cases did not fit into the above definitions of neutralization, they also were not considered examples thereof. An illustration of what is meant would be the absence of /d/ and /t/ before /l/ initially in German. This is a position in which /b/ and /p/ occur, thus providing a potential parallel. The absence of /d/ and /t/ in that position for Trubetzkoy could not be considered instances of neutralization since the sum of features shared by the pairs /p/-/t/ and /b/-/d/ would also be shared by other phonemes of the German phonological system.

In *The Linguistic School of Prague* (1966), Vachek discussed the archiphoneme concept and several problem areas encountered in its application in the Prague School. One of these areas related to the status of the sound that actually occurred in the position of neutralization. Trubetzkoy had claimed that the archiphoneme was represented in the linguistic consciousness of the speaker and hearer by the unmarked member of a correlation pair.[18] The example quoted by Vachek (p. 61) was the Russian word *zdorov'je* ("health"), where /z/ and /s/ are neutralized initially before /d/. However, /s/ was considered the unmarked member in the opposition /z/-/s/, even though it was realized as voiced in the position of neutralization. Vachek noted in this context:

> The matter was often disputed in the Prague Circle and a majority of the Prague people has never endorsed Trubetzkoy's views on the issue. Upon the whole the Prague linguists would interpret the above quoted word phonologically with the initial /zd-/ not ignoring, at the same time, the fact that the phonological opposition of the initial phoneme to its correlative partner /s/ is here neutralized . . . (p. 62)

Apparently voicing his own thoughts on the matter, Vachek noted on the archiphoneme:

> . . . any simultaneous bundle of distinctive features must be evaluated by definition as a phoneme, not as a unit subordinated to the phoneme. It appears thus that in concrete phonological structures, implemented by spoken utterances, the concept of archiphoneme has no justification. It can only be useful in structuring the phonemic systems abstracted from their implementations. And it is hardly chance that since Trubetzkoy's *Grundzüge* this term has been virtually abandoned in phonological books and papers by the Prague group. This has obviously been to its unfruitfulness.

However, subsequent developments did not support Vachek's interpretations. The usefulness of the archiphoneme concept in the representation of abstract phonological structures has been recognized in the subsequent work of generative phonologists. The archiphoneme seemed to have been "reborn" in the concept of "incompletely specified segment," although the scope of the original archiphoneme concept had changed. Incomplete feature specification now applies regardless of whether or not neutralization occurs, wherever features are predictable in any manner. Within the framework of generative theory, full feature specification within the lexicon is unnecessary and even undesirable. The predictability of features can be based on their syntagmatic or sequential co-occurrence with other features. Features are also predictable based on their paradigmatic co-occurrence, that is, based on their co-occurrence with other features in the same phonological segment. The features which can be left unspecified in generative phonology can also be more than one.

A few comments are in order here on Martinet's position on the concepts of the archiphoneme and neutralization. Martinet, who belongs to the Geneva School of linguistics, directly espoused the concepts of de Saussure and contributed to the further development of de Saussure's ideas. Martinet was exposed to a rich cross-fertilization from the Prague School of phonology and its developments. He incorporated many of its concepts into his own theories. Martinet adopted both the concepts of neutralization and of the archiphoneme and then added his own interpretations to them. In discussing the Trubetzkoyan concept of neutralization and its relation to the archiphoneme in his 1936 treatise, *Neutralisation et archiphonème*, Martinet maintained that the concepts of neutralization and archiphoneme in some instances could also be applied to disjunctive oppositions. In this same article, Martinet still made the distinction between correlations and disjunctions. Trubetzkoy had taken a similar position somewhat earlier in his 1933 *Charakter und Methode der systematischen Darstellung einer gegebenen Sprache*. However in *Die Aufhebung der phonologischen Gegensätze* (1936b), which appeared in the same issue of *Travaux du Cercle Linguistique de Prague* as Martinet's above article, Trubetzkoy had already moved away from the framework of disjunctions and correlations. There he already operated within his newly developed theory of oppositions.

Martinet never abandoned the concept of the archiphoneme. In *Éléments de linguistique générale*, published in 1960, he defined the archiphoneme as:

> . . . the sum of the relevant features common to two or more phonemes which alone present them all. (1960/1964, p. 69)

Martinet used the concept of the archiphoneme in its extended sense, including more than two phonemes.

Even though a parallel existed between the views of Trubetzkoy and Martinet linking the concept of the archiphoneme with that of neutralization, Martinet disagreed with Trubetzkoy's restricted definition of neutralization. For Martinet, neutralization could include more than two phonemes. Despite the counterexamples cited (p. 26 ff.), Martinet's conception was at variance with the basic definition of neutralization of Trubetzkoy's *Aufhebung der phonologischen Gegensätze* (1936b) and *Grundzüge der Phonologie* (1939). It is also noteworthy that Martinet adopted capital symbols as notational devices to represent the archiphoneme. Trubetzkoy had done so in the context of the morphophoneme, discussed below.

Relationship Between the Archiphoneme and the Morphophoneme

Since there are some characteristics which the archiphoneme and the morphophoneme have in common, at least in some applications, one may ask how these concepts are related historically.[19]

According to Ułaszyn (1931) it was he who coined and first used the term "morphophoneme" (*Morphonem*) in *Prace Filologiczne* (vol. XII) in 1927. He provides a full exposition of his view on the application of the concept in *Laut, Phonema, Morphonema* (1931). Ułaszyn, a linguist following the Prague School, has accepted the phoneme concept as developed by Baudouin de Courtenay (cf. p. 11 above). However, he considered his own phoneme and morphophoneme as two aspects of the Courtenayan concept of the phoneme which had been opposed to the speech sound. Ułaszyn noted:

> ... personally I feel that the concept of the phoneme is too broad and should be divided into phoneme and morphophoneme. Both of these concepts could then be contrasted with the concept of "speech sound". . . . (1931, p. 53)

For Ułaszyn the distinction between phoneme and morphoneme was one of function. He considered the phoneme as the image (*Vorstellung*) of an independent sound abstracted from sound complexes and devoid of any semantic-morphological function. He wrote:

> The phoneme is thus the image of an independent sound abstracted from sound complexes and divested of its semantic and morphological relevance. (p. 53)

A morphophoneme, on the other hand, is a phoneme in its semantic-morphological function:

> In contrast, the morphophoneme is part of a semantic, morphological element of a given language, namely of a morpheme. A morphophoneme thus is a phoneme with semantic-morphological function. (p. 53)

Phonemes, according to Ułaszyn, were to be classified according to their external relations, morphophonemes according to their internal relations. Morphophonemes thus are symbols of certain morphological relations. For example, the Polish words for "box"—*paka, pace* (plural), *paczka* (diminutive)—have the morphophonemes k-c-č(orth.cz).

Trubetzkoy adopted the term "morphophoneme" from Ułaszyn, pointing out, however, that Ułaszyn had used the concept differently, "approximately in the sense of our term phoneme" (1929c, p. 142, fn 2). Morphophonemes for Trubetzkoy referred to the alternation between two or more phonemes in the same morpheme. He called these "phoneme alternation series" (*Phonemenwechselreihen*) (p. 142):

> Since the same phoneme alternation was repeated in several morphemes, those phonemes which alternated within the same morphemes also had to be closely linked to one another. They constituted a special image in the linguistic consciousness of the speakers. We call such an image "morphophoneme," or abbreviated, "morphoneme." (1929c, p. 142)

Trubetzkoy used capital letters to denote the morphophoneme. For example, the word for "hand" in Polabian is N.Sg. rʋNkằ ~ G.Sg. rʋNħ̂ɔ ~ N.,A.,Du., rʋNcɘ (p. 142). Here Trubetzkoy used the letter *K* as the symbol for the morphophoneme. A set of rules then assigned *K* its specific value in the respective phonemes. In *Polabische Studien* (p. 142) Trubetzkoy maintained that based on their psychological content such morphonemes were "nothing more than specific 'association series' (*Assoziationsreihen)* which related to the perception of the phonological shape of a word and which lent a specific color to its individual phonemes."

In *Sur la "morphonologie"* (1929b) Trubetzkoy sketched morphophonology as separate from phonology and morphology. However, he claimed that morphophonology provided a link between the two. Morphophonology involved the study of the way in which phonological differences were used by speakers for morphological purposes. The morphophoneme was considered a "complex image" (*une idée complexe*), which could involve two or several phonemes:

> These complex images of two or more phonemes which can substitute for one another depending on the morphological context of the word, can be called morphophonemes (Trubetzkoy, 1929b/1964, p. 183)

In *Gedanken über die Morphonologie* (1931b), which appears as an appendix to *Grundzüge der Phonologie,* Trubetzkoy divided the area of morphophonology into three parts:

1. The study of the phonological structure of morphemes
2. The study of combinatory sound changes which take place in morphemes in morpheme combinations (internal sandhi)
3. The study of sound alternation series that fulfill a morphological function

With respect to the second area above, Trubetzkoy wrote in *Grundzüge:*

> This part of morphonology is not of equal importance for all languages. In certain agglutinative languages it constitutes all of morphophonology (together with the study of the phonic structure of morphemes discussed above). In certain other languages, on the other hand, it plays no role at all. (1939/1969. p. 307)

The definition of morphonology given in *Projet* essentially only covered the first of the above three categories. There, morphonology is defined as "that aspect of word phonology which deals with the phonological structure of the morphemes." The morphophoneme, in accordance with the earlier definition given in Trubetzkoy's *Sur la "morphononologie"* (1929), is defined as "a complex image of all (two or more) members of an alternation." In *Das morphonologische System der russischen Sprache* (1934) Trubetzkoy had defined the morphophoneme in essentially the same sense:

> In the linguistic consciousness of the speakers, each alternation corresponds to a morphophoneme, that is, to the morphophonological sum of all phonemes which take part in such an alternation. (p. 30)

It is of interest to note that Trubetzkoy did not use the term "morphophoneme" in *Grundzüge der Phonologie.* There morphonology is only referred to once (1939/1969, p. 240). It is somewhat misleading that his article *Gedanken über Morphonologie,* originally published in 1931 in *Travaux du Cercle linguistique de Prague* (pp. 160–163), was published posthumously as an appendix to *Grundzüge*. This tends to obscure the lack of mention of morphophonology in the body of *Grundzüge* itself. It also obscures the difference in original publication dates.

Two possible explanations might be offered to explain the absence of the morphophoneme concept and morphophonology in *Grundzüge*. According to the preface of the first German edition, Trubetzkoy had intended to add a second volume to *Grundzüge* that would have been devoted to the subject. On the other hand, much of what had been considered as part of the separate area of morphophonology in Trubetzkoy's earlier writings appears to have been covered by phonology in *Grundzüge*. For example, the study of the phonological structure of the morpheme, which had been seen as the sole purpose of morphonology in *Projet* and which constituted one of the three areas of study for morphophonology as outlined in *Gedanken über die Morphonologie*, completely shifted to phonology. In *Grundzüge* it constituted an aspect of the study of "combinatory rules" (*Kombinationslehre*) and the study of "contextual rules" (*Abgrenzungslehre*).

> . . . combinatory rules always presuppose a higher phonological unit within the framework of which they are valid. But this higher phonological unit need not always be a word. In many languages not the word . . . but the morpheme must be regarded as such a unit. . . . the first task of any investigation of combinations is merely to determine the phonological unit within which combinatory rules can be studied most appropriately. The second task is the division of the "frame units" (words or morphemes) with respect to their phonological structure. (1939/1969, p. 249)

Ďurovič (1967), who called attention to Trubetzkoy's lack of treatment of morphophonology in *Grundzüge*, suggested that Trubetzkoy may have given up the idea of morphonology altogether, or that he may have intended a chapter on morphonology in a limited sense so as to include only free morpheme alternations.

From what has been said it is apparent that the concepts of the archiphoneme and the morphophoneme had separate and different origins and, at one time, were separate entities. The archiphoneme, like the phoneme, was a phonological unit. The morphophoneme was a functional unit that belonged to the separate area of morphophonemics.

As can be surmised, the phonological contrasts involved in the archiphonemes and those found in morpheme alternations were not always mutually exclusive. Some such phonological contrasts could always be viewed in terms of the archiphoneme as well as in terms of the morphophoneme. In fact, in discussing the archiphoneme, Jakobson had noted in *Remarques* that:

> ... the grammatical alternation of two members of an opposition (that is, the morphological use of this opposition) could be an important concomitant factor which may aid in separating the common base from the dividing characteristic [*principium divisionis*]. (Jakobson, 1929/1962, p. 9)

For example, an archiphoneme is posited in the case of German syllable-final neutralization of voiced obstruents, e.g., dīp, hʊnt, tāk (thief, dog, day). However, when the respective phonological contrast is viewed in terms of a morpheme alternation a morphophoneme can be posited as well. The following illustration represents a case where the archiphoneme and the morphophoneme do not coalesce. Neutralization is assumed in English in cases of sound sequences where a voiceless sibilant occurs before a voiceless obstruent in word-initial position. The voiceless sibilant is then considered as the representation of an underlying archiphoneme for the contrast /s/-/z/. In this case there can be no question of a morphophoneme since no morphemic alternation is involved. Neutralization and the resultant archiphoneme usually involved a two-way contrast. This was not necessarily true for morphophophonemic contrasts, which could be larger.

It appears that, originally, morphological alternations were viewed as support for an archiphoneme in the case of automatic alternations (cf. the above quote from Jakobson's 1929 article). Despite the fact that Trubetzkoy in his earlier writings, had developed the idea that morphophonology constituted a separate area of study, in his culminating work, *Grundzüge*, a large aspect of morphophonology was actually considered within the framework of phonology. The morphophoneme thus coalesced, at least partially, with the archiphoneme.

In American linguistics, Leonard Bloomfield, in *Menomini Morphophonemics* (1939), adopted the concept of the morphophoneme, as did others. However, Bloomfield added a different emphasis. He distinguished between internal sandhi or morphophonemes and morphological variation. He wrote:

> The process of description leads us to set up each morphological element in a theoretical basic form and then to state the deviations from this basic form which appear when this element is combined with other elements. (1939/1970, p. 352)

Bloomfield further specified for his examples that the derivative statements were to be ordered.

Trubetzkoy claimed that in the linguistic consciousness of the speaker each alternation corresponds to a morphophoneme, that is, to a morphonological unit consisting of the sum of phonemes involved in the alternation. He also used abstract symbols for the representation of the morphophoneme. However, he did not quite speak of a theoretical basic form. It was the conceptualization of the morphophoneme in terms of a theoretical basic form which had appealed to the generative phonologists. The concept was first adopted and further developed by Morris Halle in *The Sound Pattern of Russian* (1959).

The Concept of Markedness in Generative Phonology: Its Origins and Use in Prague Phonology

Markedness was another concept introduced into generative theory. It was closely related to the concept of naturalness, which had made its appearance in generative phonology with Halle's introduction of natural classes into phonology. Halle specifically dealt with this notion in his work, *Phonology in Generative Grammar* (1962).

The notion of markedness in generative phonology was based on the rediscovery of the Praguian marked and unmarked values for features. Chomsky and Halle, in *The Sound Pattern of English* (1968), argued that their earlier account of phonological descriptions had not made use of the "intrinsic" content of features. The concept of markedness appeared to them suitable to express certain general observations about language that could not be represented in the earlier framework. These included the observation that some features have a higher expectancy or generality of occurrence in language in general as well as in individual languages. They noted that there were features which were somehow preferred. The concept of markedness also appeared useful in distinguishing feature values which were "normal" or "natural" from features values which were "less natural" and "less normal." By utilizing the concept of markedness Chomsky and Halle hoped to bring out these distinctions and to make a phonological description explanatory on a deeper level than could have been done within the earlier framework. The notion that a feature value was more natural or normal in a given environment than its opposite value applies to the sequential (syntagmatic) as well as the segmental (paradigmatic) context of the feature in question. Normal or natural was equated with the unmarked value of a feature. That which was less normal or less expected or general was the marked value of a given feature.

In the earlier framework, it had not been possible to express such observations about language. Support for what is normal or natural and thus unmarked was sought from such diverse sources as ease of production, language typology, language change, language pathology, and language acquisition. Ease of production would indicate assignment of an unmarked value, for example. In language acquisition unmarked values were thought to be acquired first, and unmarked values were also thought to be lost last in aphasia.[20] A potential conflict arose, for example, in language acquisition, where the bilabial nasal "m" tends to be acquired first and accordingly should be considered as unmarked. However, on the basis of generality of occurrence, not "m" but "n" should be considered the unmarked member of the nasal contrast /m/-/n/. The concept of naturalness is also closely linked to the assumption that underlying any phonological system is a universal phonological structure.

Implicit in the assumption that some segments, features, and feature combinations are more normal, natural, and preferrred, is the idea that that which is normal, natural, and preferred is also less complex. Conversely, that which is less normal, less natural, and less preferred is seen as more complex. Complexity in generative phonology is viewed in terms of speech production (perception?) as well as in terms of providing an evaluation criterion for grammar, where the most highly valued grammar is also the least complex.

The concept of markedness thus became formally linked with the criterion of simplicity in the evaluation metric of a grammar: a segment is considered less complex, hence more natural (and thus preferable), the fewer marked and the more unmarked features it has. In the earlier feature framework used in generative phonology before the advent of the markedness concept, a dictionary entry consisted of a distinctive feature matrix which contained three types of phonological entries: +, −, and 0. Based on the criterion of simplicity, + and − were considered as having "equal cost" while the zeros had no cost, representing the predictable elements which were subsequently filled in by morpheme structure rules.

According to Chomsky and Halle, the major difference between the earlier Praguian conception of markedness, especially as developed by Trubetzkoy and by them, is that in the earlier Praguian conception the "marked co-efficient of a feature was assumed always to be + and the unmarked co-efficient always −" (1968, p. 404). However, the discussion below points out differences. According to Chomksy and Halle such an assumption placed serious restrictions on the usefulness of the markedness concept. In this context they stated:

> ... this restriction loses force unless it is coupled with the assumption of a fixed set of phonological features so that it is impossible to replace in the description of a particular language a given feature by its complement—for example, the feature "tense" by "lax," "voice" by "voicelessness" or "rounding" by "unroundedness." (p. 404)

They go on to say that, without this further assumption:

> ... the proposal concerning the relationship between marked and positively specified features is weakened, but it is still stronger than the position taken here since it does not permit the marked value of a particular feature to depend on a particular context. (p. 404)

Chomsky and Halle (1968) refined and adopted the earlier concept of markedness to suit their own use. They introduced the notational devices M and U for the marked and unmarked specification of a feature respectively. In their use of the concept in *The Sound Pattern of English,* the marked coefficient of a feature now is no longer linked with the + co-efficient of a feature and the unmarked value with the − co-efficient. The new framework also dispensed with the earlier 0 notation, which was no longer required.

In the new framework of distinctive features, which now formally includes the concept of markedness, a dictionary representation consists of two levels. The first level is a deeper, more abstract, explanatory level. Matrices consist for the most part of marked and unmarked values, and only the marked values have weight complexity; the unmarked values cost nothing. In this model, both predictability and naturalness are lumped together and represented by the unmarked values. A set of universal, language-independent rules then translates the U-M matrices into a second, less abstract, language-specific set of matrices. At this level, each square is filled in either by a + or a − entry. The zeros of the earlier framework are submersed into the U values of the new framework. They have no more overt function in the second set of matrices, and consequently they have been dropped (see Chomsky and Halle, 1968, table 12 (p. 412) and table 14 (p. 415)).

To make markedness theory work, it is of course important to discover what is marked and what is unmarked in a given environment and to find the correct set of universal rules to plot these values into language-specific +/− matrices. At times there may also be a problem in determining what is to be considered natural, since naturalness can be considered from various points of view. A distinction may also have to be made between what is considered natural from a universal point of view and what is considered natural within a particular language. It would seem that the concept of markedness, as it exists in its current form in generative theory, should be taken as a proposal that awaits a great deal of further thought and exploration.

After this cursory summary of current markedness theory, we may now ask how the concept originated and was used in the Prague School, and what its revived form still has in common with its origins.

Origin of the Term "Markedness"   Since the notion of markedness was a concept that first appeared in the linguistic literature in German, it is helpful to know what the term meant in German and how it was originally used.

The term "markedness" is a translation of the German *merkmalhaltig. Merkmalhaltig* ("containing a mark or characteristic") and *merkmaltragend* ("carrying a mark or a characteristic or feature) are derived from the noun *Merkmal*. In Prague phonology the term *Merkmal* was used synonymously with *phonologische Eigenschaft* ("phonological or distinctive property"). Jakobson adopted the English term "distinctive feature" for *Merkmal* when he first brought his *Merkmalanalyse* ("feature analysis") to the United States. A second translation equivalent for *Merkmal* is found in the context of *Korrelation* ("correlation") and subsequently also in the context of opposition. The term *Merkmal* in this context is rendered as "mark."[21]

The concept of *Korrelationsmerkmal* ("correlation mark") represented a very important notion for both the history of distinctive features and the original concept of markedness. Terminologically, it seems that in this context "mark" was taken into English via the French term *marque,* a term borrowed from metrics, as were the terms "marked" and "unmarked" (*marqué* and *non-marqué*, respectively). The French *marque* in this context had been adopted from a work on metrics by Verrier on a suggestion by Roman Jakobson.[22]

Marque de correlation ("correlation mark") is defined in *Projet de terminologie phonologique standardisée*, (1931) as a "sound element which, opposed to its absence, forms a correlation mark."[23] The adjectives *merkmalhaltig* and *merkmallos* thus originally meant "having a feature" and "not having a feature," respectively, or, when used in the context of correlation, "marked" and "unmarked." Their definitions are contained in "marked correlative series" (*série corrélative marquée*), defined in *Projet* as a "correlative series which is characterized by the presence of a correlation mark." An "unmarked correlative series" (*série corrélative non-marquée*) was defined as "a correlation series which is characterized by the absence of the correlation mark."

It becomes apparent that ultimately two separate, though related, concepts developed from the underlying German term *Merkmal*, depending on the context in which the term was used. The coefficients of *Merkmal* when used in the context of distinctive feature were + and −, in the context of correlation, *marked* and *unmarked*.

As shown below, the relationship between these respective values (+, *marked*; −, *unmarked*) was not isomorphic. Even in their original use, the terms "marked" and "unmarked" could not always be considered identical with the plus and minus values of the distinctive features as claimed by Chomsky and Halle, who maintained that:

> A major difference between the Praguian conception of markedness and our own is that in the former the marked coefficient of the feature was assumed always to be + and the unmarked coefficient always to be −. (1968, p. 404)

Origin of the Concept "Markedness"   It may be safe to claim that a fully developed theory of markedness did not exist in Prague phonology. The concept itself first arose in the context of the theory of correlations. Markedness originally was only secondarily associated with neutralization. It was linked in the first place with the concept of the archiphoneme.

As noted earlier (p. 4), the concept of correlation was initially defined by Jakobson, Karcevskij, and Trubetzkoy in the 1928 *Proposition au Premier Congrès International de Linguistes,* as follows:

> . . . a phonological correlation consists of a set of binary oppositions
> defined by a common principle which can be thought of independent
> of each pair of opposing members. (1928/1962, p. 3)

Abstracted and thought of independently, this common principle *(principe commun)* formed the basis for the subsequent distinctive feature theory. In conjunction with correlation, the common principle was to become the correlation mark and form the basis for the marked versus unmarked dichotomy.

According to Jakobson, and as can be surmised from the pertinent literature, Trubetzkoy was the first to develop the concept of markedness. However, Jakobson subsequently expanded the concept to apply to morphology and semantics as well. (Cf. Jakobson, *Zur Struktur des russischen Verbums,* 1932a, and his *Beitrag zur allgemeinen Kasuslehre,* 1936a.)

Trubetzkoy made the first mention of markedness in *Die phonologischen Systeme* (1931a), where he maintained that two members of a correlative opposition did not have equal weight *(gleichberechtigt sein)*:

> . . . the one member has the particular property or has it in its positive
> form, the other does not have it or has it in its negative form. We
> designate the former as *marked,* the latter as *unmarked.* (p. 97)

The relationship between such correlative oppositions as rounded/unrounded and voiced/voiceless was here also seen as one of active affirmation as contrasted with passive negation of a property. In this context, it is justified to consider marked as the plus and unmarked as the minus coefficient of a property or feature.

In *Die Konsonantensysteme der ostkaukasischen Sprachen* (1931e), Trubetzkoy again used the term "active" in the sense of marked and "passive" in the sense of unmarked. The passive or unmarked values of the oppositions voiced/voiceless, glottal/nonglottal, and spirant/stop for the East Caucasian obstruent systems were given as voiceless, nonglottal, and occlusive.

Trubetzkoy insisted that every phonological description had to contain a specification of what was to be considered as marked and unmarked for the system which was being described. In *Die Konsonantensysteme der ostkaukasischen Sprachen* he intimated how this should be done. In a less detailed phonological description only the marked correlative properties needed to be specified. Rules could then further specify the conditions under which both marked and unmarked properties occurred in that language:

In a less detailed transcription only the active correlative properties need to be specified. However, in describing a language, the conditions of occurrence for both unmarked and marked properties must be indicated. (Trubetzkoy, 1931e, p. 15)

Instructions for the way in which marked and unmarked values of a correlative opposition were to be indicated in actual transcription were given by Trubetzkoy in *Principes de transcription phonologique* (1931d). He suggested the symbol ‿ for unmarked and the symbol ⁀ for marked. The section dealing with markedness is not quite clear. However, it appears that Trubetzkoy was proposing a two-level notation of markedness: the symbols ‿ and ⁀ occurring at the bottom lower right of a phoneme seemed to indicate the "natural" or "predetermined" value of a segment as marked or unmarked. A notation that appeared at the top right of the phoneme, in addition to the notation at the lower level, indicated the behavior of the segments with respect to marking in morphological alternation. In other words, it indicated the value a particular segment assumes in the particular context where it alternates with its "natural" or "predetermined value." Trubetzkoy did not state how to choose a segment as marked or unmarked although he regarded it as an important question. It was also a matter on which he subsequently changed his mind.

The decision as to what was to be considered as unmarked or marked was originally left to the linguistic consciousness of the speaker. For example, in *Die phonologischen Systeme,* Trubetzkoy noted:

This [markedness] is not at all arbitrary. In each and every instance, the average member of the particular linguistic community will make a decision in the same direction. (1931a, p. 98)

It would seem, however, that the linguistic consciousness of speakers may differ from language to language since it is likely to be conditioned by one's mother tongue. The judgment about what is marked and unmarked may therefore also differ from language to language.

Trubetzkoy actually gave some examples which would make this point. In the voiced/voiceless opposition of stops, a native Russian speaker considers the voiceless members as unmarked and the voiced members as marked, while for a North German the opposite would be true.[24]

In *La phonologie actuelle* (1933a) Trubetzkoy again made a statement with respect to markedness: ". . . it is only phonological consciousness which can guide us." However, here Trubetzkoy was elaborating on what he meant by phonological consciousness. A normal native speaker has no notion of what is marked and what is unmarked, although he or she will intuitively feel that, for example, between the three phonemes /p/, /b/, and aspirated /p'/, /p/ is the simplest and most normal phoneme which is free from any secondary quality. The /p/ is therefore to be regarded as unmarked.

The idea of what is most normal and least complex also appears in *Die Konsonantensysteme der ostkaukasischen Sprachen* (1931e). In *Grundzüge* (1939/1969) normalcy was also coupled with naturalness from the point of view of articulation:

> In any correlation . . . a "natural absence of marking" is attributed to that opposition member whose production requires the least deviation from normal breathing. (1939/1969, p. 146)

Based on this "natural" point of view Trubetzkoy then considered the fortis consonant the marked member of the correlation of tension fortis/lenis.

A similar view on least complexity was also expressed by Jakobson in *On Ancient Greek Prosody*:

> A marked category tends to be interpreted in relation to the unmarked one as a compound, complex category opposed to a simple one. (1937/1962, p. 266)

Trubetzkoy maintained that decisions as to which phonemes should be considered marked and unmarked values can also find psychological support. An example would be the directions in which children make mistakes. However, it is important to stress that what Trubetzkoy considered as marked and unmarked was not synonymous with what Jakobson subsequently designated by + and − in his feature system. Some of the differences that emerge include the following:

1. The features which were marked and unmarked could differ from language to language in the Trubetzkoyan conception
2. Although the "surface" value of a feature could be marked, a segment could still be interpreted as having an underlying unmarked value

For example, with respect to the first difference Trubetzkoy maintained that in the case of the oppositions of timbre *(Eigentongegensätze)* not every language of the East Caucasian group considered the same correlation member as marked (Table 1). Trubetzkoy gave other examples where the +/− coefficients of

Table 1.   Opposition of timbre—light/dark *(hell/dunkel)*—in East Caucasian languages

Group A		Group B	
Light	Dark	Light	Dark
Passive	Active	Active	Passive
Normal	Elongated resonance cavity	Shortened resonance cavity	Normal
Unrounded	Rounded	Emphasized palatalization	Nonpalatalization
Marked	Unmarked	Marked	Unmarked

marked and unmarked change depending on the language, for example, vowel quantity in German and Czech.

With respect to the second difference noted above, Trubetzkoy maintained that the coefficients of a marked and unmarked property can change, if they are predictable. He stated in *Die phonologischen Systeme*:

> In those positions where the correlative property of a phoneme loses its phonological relevance, *the phoneme in question is identified with the unmarked correlation member, even though it may in fact be identical with the marked correlation member.* (1931a, p. 98; emphasis added)

The example cited by Trubetzkoy was palatalization of Russian consonants when they occur before other palatal consonants. Even though such consonants are "objectively marked as palatalized," they are nevertheless identified with the unmarked value: śt'inà (wall), śveček'ə (candle), where the ś (marked) is identified with s (unmarked). A further example is that of the accented and unaccented vowels in Russian. Trubetzkoy maintained that, based on his linguistic consciousness, a Russian speaker will regard the accented vowels as unmarked. It seems to be implied, though Trubetzkoy does not say so explicitly, that the unaccented vowels are predictable from the accented vowels, but not vice versa. In the case of palatalization in Russian, the "surface" + value is nevertheless identified with the unmarked value.

Trubetzkoy also distinguished between the representative of the archiphoneme and the symbol for the archiphoneme: the symbol for the archiphoneme is that unit which occurs in the linguistic consciousness of every speaker. It is always unmarked. In contrast, the representative of an archiphoneme is that unit which actually occurs in a particular position. It may either be marked or unmarked. If it is predictable, it must be identified with the unmarked value.

The distinction between the representative and the symbol of an archiphoneme was eliminated in *Anleitung zu phonologischen Beschreibungen* (1935), where marking was explicitly associated with neutralization. The unmarked form now was always that segment which appeared as the sole representative of the archiphoneme in positions where a particular contrast had been neutralized.

This could be illustrated by an example from German. Trubetzkoy considered the German long vowels unmarked in the opposition of vowel quantity because they occurred in the position of neutralization. In contrast, short vowels were considered marked because they did not occur in the position of neutralization. For Czech, on the other hand, Trubetzkoy considered the short vowels unmarked because they appear in the position of neutralization. Position of neutralization rather than the speaker's linguistic consciousness or intuition thus constituted a formal criterion for determining the unmarked status of a segment. A reminder of earlier references to the speaker's linguistic consciousness and the distinction between archiphoneme symbol and representative was seen in cases of assimilation. In instances of assimilation a segment could appear as marked but was identified with its unmarked value.

As soon as the concept of neutralization became linked to markedness, its application and the determination of marked and unmarked values became restricted and more difficult. In *Die Aufhebung der phonologischen Gegensätze* (1936b) Trubetzkoy went one step further and explicitly restricted the use of the markedness concept to those oppositions which could be neutralized. The following illustrates the position of neutralizable oppositions in the Trubetzkoyan classification (cf. Table 1):

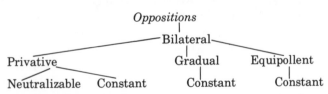

Cases of conflict arose in determining markedness based on the criterion of position of neutralization. These were instances in which different positions of neutralization were also associated with different representatives of the archiphoneme. In such instances the opposition member to be considered unmarked was the one that occurred in the *most normal position*.

By making the selection of an unmarked member dependent on its occurrence in the position of neutralization, frequency became an additional corollary of markedness. Trubetzkoy was quite aware of this. In *Grundzüge* (1939/1969, p. 262), Zipf's law was restated to denote this general tendency:

1. Zipf's law: the less complicated the realization of a phoneme, the greater its frequency.
2. Trubetzkoy: of the two members of a privative opposition the unmarked member occurs more frequently in continuous speech than the marked member

Comparison with Current Markedness Theory   In comparison with today's version, markedness for Trubetzkoy was severely restricted by the very framework of his theory. The concept only applied to certain oppositions: originally to correlations, and subsequently to privative (neutralizable) oppositions, that is, to oppositions characterized by the presence versus the absence of a feature. Marking comprised neither the equipollent nor the gradual oppositions of his classification. As demonstrated later in this text, both these types of oppositions were subsequently also transformed to privative oppositions in the framework of the Jakobsonian distinctive features and included in the + and − notation. Theoretically, they thus also became available for inclusion in the marked-unmarked dichotomy.

It is also clear that today's version of markedness theory is much wider in scope in other respects as well. It appears that Trubetzkoy had only incidentally linked the notion of markedness and naturalness from a language-universal point of view. All his arguments for the concept of markedness were language specific. However, certain implications for language-universal arguments were not lacking, for example, his observation that certain rules for neutralization probably underlie all languages, and his arguments for what is simplest and most normal in determining marked and unmarked values. His argument involving simplicity and normalcy was marred, however, by his allusions to speaker's linguistic consciousness. To rely on a speaker's linguistic consciousness would certainly slant what is considered normal and simple since judgments based on linguistic consciousness would almost certainly tend to be language dependent.

Psychological terminology aside, marking for Trubetzkoy was determined above all by the overall functioning of the phonological system and by the role the individual oppositions played in a given language. Accordingly, marking was a relative concept since these were matters which varied from language to language.

It is noteworthy to point out that some contradiction arose as a result of Trubetzkoy's shift from his earlier version to his subsequent view restricted by neutralization. The following example illustrates the point. If the unmarked value was determined by position of neutralization only, then the unaccented vowels in Russian would have to be considered as unmarked. This was clearly not the case. It was shown earlier that the accented vowels were considered unmarked, since they were predictable from the accented vowels. What needed to be distinguished was the notion of simplicity or naturalness in terms of segment structure and in terms of phonological function. In terms of segment structure, the unmarked member was the opposition member which was free from any secondary quality (see p. 64). In terms of phonological function, the unmarked member was the one which occurred in the position of neutralization.

Simplicity from a segment-structure point of view may thus differ from simplicity based on phonological function. For example, vowel length seems to be marked in regard to segment structure, that is, vowel plus a feature of length. This is actually the case in Czech, where the marked value, based on segment structure criteria, also coincides with the marked value based on phonological function. In German, on the other hand, even though vowel quantity is associated with the same segment structure complexity, it must be considered unmarked from the point of view of the phonological system since it appears in the position of neutralization. Likewise, stressed vowels in Russian seem to be marked according to segment complexity, although in phonological function they must be considered unmarked.

Consideration of all aspects of the theory of markedness leads to the conclusion that Trubetzkoy's original concept of markedness resembled today's version more closely than his subsequent, modified, and more restricted conception in which neutralization became the decisive factor.

RELATIONSHIP OF THE DISTINCTIVE FEATURE
CONCEPT TO PHONETICS AND PHONOLOGY
IN GENERATIVE GRAMMAR AND IN PRAGUE PHONOLOGY

The relationship between phonetics and phonology, as viewed in the early Prague days and as it stands within the current generative framework, relates directly to distinctive feature theory. In the generative framework the function of the phonological component was defined as follows:

> The major function of the phonological component is to derive the phonetic representation of an utterance from the surface structure assigned to it by the syntactic component, that is, from its representation in terms of classificatory features of the lexical items it contains, its other nonlexical formatives, and its analysis in terms of immediate constituents, all of this material having been modified in an appropriate way by the readjustment rules. (Chomsky and Halle, 1968, p. 63)

Below we will discuss how this statement is related to an earlier discussed conception, that of de Saussure.

De Saussure (1916) divided language into *langue* and *parole*.[25] Following de Saussure, Trubetzkoy in *Grundzüge* divided the study of sounds *(Lautlehre)* into one study related to *parole,* that is, phonetics, and into one study related to *langue,* that is, phonology (1939/1969, p. 3 ff.) Phonetics was to deal with the physical aspects of sounds and phonology with relations, functions, and values, since *langue* also dealt with social norms.[26]

De Saussure himself had not as yet insisted on a division between two kinds of sound study. The Polish scholar Baudouin de Courtenay apparently was the first to make such a distinction, in *Versuch einer Theorie phonetischer Alternationen* (1895). He differentiated between "psychophonetics" and "physiophonetics." This terminology was subsequently criticized and later replaced by phonology and phonetics. However, the distinction between the two approaches to speech sounds did not make any headway until after 1928 and the programmatic *Thèses presentées au premier Congrès des philologues slaves.* It is also of interest that at the First International Congress of Linguists held in The Hague in that year, the term "phonology" was not mentioned even once. However, at that Congress, a short program was presented by the three Russian scholars, R. Jakobson, N.S. Trubetzkoy, and S. Karcesvkij, in which the distinction between the study of sounds pertaining to the speech act *(parole)* and the study of sound pertaining to the system of language *(langue)* was set forth. The term "phonology" appeared for the first time in the new sense which had been given to it by the Prague School in 1929[27] in the first two volumes of the *Travaux du Cercle linguistique de Prague.* By 1930, an International Association for Phonological Studies was founded with Trubetzkoy as its president; and at the Second International Congress of Linguists in Geneva, 1931, one plenary session was for the first time devoted to phonology.

The Prague School division of *Lautlehre* ("study of sounds") into phonetics and phonology was based on the following rationale, which Trubetzkoy as well as Jakobson adhered to throughout: phonetics and phonology were oriented toward different goals; phonetics was concerned with the physical aspect and phonology with the functional aspect of sounds. Therefore, since phonetics dealt with physical phenomena, the methods of the natural sciences applied to its study. Since phonology was concerned with sounds as social norms, the methods of the social sciences applied. However, in the early Praguian expositions on phonology and phonetics it was never made clear what was meant by either of these methods or wherein the distinction lay. Nor has such a distinction ever been made in the practice of linguistics anywhere.

However, Trubetzkoy drew an unwarranted conclusion with respect to the above division of phonetics and phonology. Linguistics is only interested in the functional, relational aspects of language, that is, in *langue.* Phonetics therefore is only an ancillary science and not part of linguistics proper. For this reason Trubetzkoy maintained that these two approaches should be kept separate in theory as well as in practice. Trubetzkoy adhered to this distinction throughout his career, although he did not want to completely cut the ties between the two. He considered a resynthesis of phonology and phonetics whenever phonological concepts were of help in the segmentation of the speech continuum so that he could arrive at "typical articulatory positions" and "typical sounds" in his descriptions of the sound continuum. Trubetzkoy also considered it reasonable that phonetic terminology be used for phonological studies. Furthermore, phonetic transcription served as a basis for the discovery of the distinctive sound oppositions in a given language, that is, of its phonemes. Trubetzkoy maintained, however, that on the "higher" levels of phonological description, phonology should be considered independently of phonetics.

The viewpoint that phonetics lies outside of linguistics proper is, of course, quite alien to generative phonology, as is the distinction beween the two separate methods suggested for the study of phonetics and phonology.

For Trubetzkoy the scope of phonology extended to the determination of the phonemic inventory of a language, the analysis of the structure of the phoneme system including phoneme combinations, relative phoneme frequency, the discovery and description of the characterology of a system, and the search for universal laws which govern any of the above areas. In generative phonology the ultimate objectives of study are somewhat different. Even though it is necessary to have the results of some of the above endeavors as input, they are taken for granted and the concern is not with their discovery. The phonological component of a grammar within the generative framework focuses on the conversion of these higher phonological units to their ultimate phonetic equivalents.

It develops that the objectives to be met by the phonological component have a direct effect on the fate of the concept of the distinctive feature since the generative framework distinguishes between features whose values are different on the phonological level and the phonetic level. The relationship is one of binary classificatory and n-ary phonetic features. Throughout the development of feature analysis, features, when binary, were binary phonologically and phonetically. When they were considered nonbinary, they were nonbinary in terms of phonology and phonetics. The distinction between phonology and phonetics had never been one of binarity versus nonbinarity, but one between distinctiveness and nondistinctiveness, or between phonological relevancy and nonrelevancy. The relationship between binary, classificatory, and n-ary phonetic features thus is a wholly new one established in generative phonology.[28]

A FIRST UNIFIED THEORY OF OPPOSITIONS

From a historical viewpoint the development of distinctive feature theory raises the following series of questions:

1. How and where did the idea of such a unit develop? How did it fit into the development of phonological theory? What was its relationship to the most closely related concepts in this development?

2. After the theoretical establishment of such a unit, and after the phoneme had been defined as a "bundle of distinctive features," what were the developments which contributed to an actual final breakdown of the phoneme into its ultimate components? What is the relationship of these features, after they have been isolated, to each other? What can be said about the nature of these features?

The questions under (1) have been treated in the preceding sections. Regarding the questions raised under (2), already mentioned is that within the framework of correlations and disjunctions an analysis of phoneme relationships was fairly restricted. Even after the definition of the phoneme had evolved into a "bundle of distinctive features," distinctive features were not immediately accessible to abstraction. Isolating features in their ultimate form involved a relatively protracted history. This development is traced below.

Trubetzkoy was the first to replace the old dichotomy of correlations and disjunctions in the initial classification of oppositions, recognizing its inadequacy. He developed a more complex classification that took into account additional distinctions and also revealed different types of oppositive relationships. He felt that these relationships held the key to the degree of coherence, symmetry, and equilibrium that a phonological system should possess. The development of his classification and its ultimate appearance in *Grundzüge* are summarized below.

Trubetzkoy's scheme of oppositions appeared first in *Essai d'une théorie des oppositions phonologiques* (1936c), where he proposed a new set of oppositive distinctions.

Vachek, as mentioned earlier, was a chronicler of overall Praguian development. He (1966) pointed out that Trubetzkoy had succeeded, in his new classification, in bringing out finer distinctions lacking in the earlier framework. He further drew attention to additional insights that flowed from Trubetzkoy's work and paved the way for the ultimate developments in distinctive feature theory. To quote, Vachek maintained that:

> . . . the establishment of different categories of mutual phonemic relations clearly implied the focusing of attention on different, so far unnoticed aspects of the classified phonemes . . . thus it could but strengthen the conception of the phoneme as a bundle of distinctive features and indirectly prepare the way for Jakobson's and Halle's theory of the binary oppositions of distinctive features composing the phonemes. (1966, p.58)

Summary of the New Classification of Oppositions

In both *Essai d'une théorie des oppositions phonologiques* (1936c) and *Grundzüge der Phonologie* (1939/1969) Trubetzkoy proposed a basic distinction between two types of oppositions which he called bilateral and multilateral.[29]

Bilateral oppositions consisted of pairs of phonemes in which the sum of shared features was common to the two members of that opposition only, for example, /t/-/d/ and /m/-/b/ in German and English.

Multilateral oppositions consisted of phoneme pairs in which the sum of shared features also was found in other phonemes of the same system, for example, /p/-/t/ in English and German. The common features of this phoneme pair also occur in /k/.

The second distinction made by Trubetzkoy was between proportional and isolated oppositions. *Proportional oppositions* consisted of phoneme pairs in which the relationship between its members was repeated in other phoneme pairs of the same system. *Isolated oppositions* consisted of phoneme pairs in which the relationship between its members was not repeated in any other phoneme pair of the same system. Table 2 illustrates these distinctions.

The distinction between bilateral and multilateral oppositions was considered extremely important by Trubetzkoy. Not all phonemes could participate in bilateral oppositions (for example, German /h/). Trubetzkoy noted that multilateral oppositions al-

Table 2. Oppositions (examples are given from German)

	Bilateral	Multilateral
Proportional	t-d : p-b : s-z	p-t : b-d : m-n
Isolated	r-l	f-z

ways outnumber bilateral oppositions. Also, proportional oppositions are always in a minority in any system, but the numerical
ratio between proportional and isolated oppositions varies.
Trubetzkoy considered proportional oppositions the most important ones.[30]

Trubetzkoy further divided bilateral oppositions into *neutralizable* and *constant oppositions*. The distinction between the
two, according to Trubetzkoy, also represents a tremendous
psychological difference. The relationship between the members
of a neutralizable opposition was judged to be closer and more
"intimate" than that between two constant opposition members.[31]
Trubetzkoy considered each member of a neutralizable opposition
an "archiphoneme plus a specific property." This interpretation
even applied to those positions where all features of such an opposition were phonologically relevant. For the constant oppositions he found it more difficult to abstract the archiphoneme, that
is, the features shared by the members of such an opposition.[32]

In *Essai d'une théorie* as well as in *Grundzüge* Trubetzkoy
divided multilateral oppositions into homogeneous and
heterogeneous oppositions. *Homogeneous oppositions* were
phoneme pairs which could be thought of as the outermost points
in a chain made up of bilateral oppositions. An example is the
phoneme pair /u/-/e/ in German, where the only feature shared
was that of vocality, a feature common to all vowels. /u/ and
/e/ were connected as the outermost points in a chain as follows:
/u/-/o/, /o/-/ö/, /ö/-/e/. Similarly, the pair /n/-/ŋ/ was connected as
follows: /x/-/k/, /k/-/g/, /g/-/ŋ/. *Heterogeneous oppositions* consisted
of phoneme pairs which could not be thought of in terms of chains
of bilaterally related phoneme pairs or in terms of a bilateral
contrast to each other, for example, the phonemes /p/ and /t/ in
German and English.

Trubetzkoy discovered that heterogeneous relations occur
more frequently than homogeneous relations in any given system
but that homogeneous relations play a more important role for
the specification of the phonological system. Expanding his classificatory scheme even further, Trubetzkoy divided homogeneous
oppositions into linear and nonlinear oppositions.[33]

Linear oppositions consisted of phoneme pairs in which there
was only one possible chain through which the phoneme pair
could be linked. An example is the phoneme pair /x/-/ŋ/ in German
which, according to Trubetzkoy, could only be linked as follows:
/x-k, k-g, g-ŋ/. *Nonlinear oppositions* were phoneme pairs in which

there was more than one possible chain. An example is the German phoneme pair /u/-/e/. The following chains are possible: /u-o-ö-e/, /u-ü-ö-e, /u-ü-i-e/, and /u-o-a-ä-e/.

Figure 1 summarizes Trubetzkoy's reclassification of oppositions. It provides several types of information and distinctions based on several different types of criteria, discussed below.[34]

The division between multilateral and bilateral oppositions is a distinction based on the transparency or opacity of opposition relationships. Bilateral oppositions were those in which the phonemes are distinguished solely on the basis of one property or feature; this is not the case for multilateral oppositions.

The distinction between isolated and proportional oppositions, on the other hand, is based on a frequency ratio and comprises both multilateral and bilateral oppositions.

The distinction between neutralizable and constant oppositions only applies to bilateral oppositions. It is based on distributional criteria or contextual constraints.

The distinction between homogeneous and heterogeneous oppositions applies to multilateral oppositions and appears to have as its basis the insight that, at least with respect to homogeneous oppositions, opposition complexity can be further analyzed and broken down in nonarbitrary ways.

This last distinction is theoretically important and seems to have carried phonological analysis one step further toward the analysis of the phonological system into a finite set of distinctive

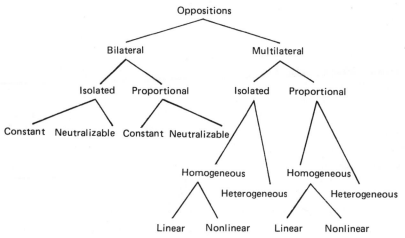

Figure 1. Trubetzkoy's reclassification of oppositions.

features. Trubetzkoy seemed to have discovered through his analysis that with the exception of heterogeneous relations multilateral oppositions were convertible into a series of bilateral relationships. For example, in English the multilateral opposition /p/-/z/ can be interpreted as the following series of bilateral oppositions: /p/-/t/, /t/-/s/, /s/-/z/. The distinction between linear and nonlinear oppositions referred to the obligatory nature of chaining. In the case of linear oppositions, according to Trubetzkoy, there was no choice in chaining when they were broken down into bilateral oppositions. This was not true for nonlinear oppositions, where a limited number of such choices exists. Homogeneous relations could thus be thought of as a "deck" of bilateral relations. In the case of linear oppositions, only one chain was possible. In the case of nonlinear oppositions a limited number of alternate chains was possible. Homogeneous relations clearly seemed to relate to the idea of feature hierarchy. In the case of nonlinear oppositions, several possible choices were available within the structure of the phonological system. In both instances, however, the choice was not arbitrary.

Multilateral homogeneous relations could thus be easily converted into a chain of bilateral relations. It was then possible to view the degree of closeness or relatedness between the members of a multilateral opposition in terms of respective points in a hierarchy established by this conversion procedure.

The relations which remained nontransparent or opaque for Trubetzkoy were those which he called multilateral heterogeneous relations. These were always more numerous than the homogeneous ones.

At this point it would be helpful to call attention to a fine distinction between the Trubetzkoyan term "bilateral" and the Jakobsonian term "binary." In the Trubetzkoyan classification, the determination of what is bilateral was based on the common core of an opposition, that is, of two phonemes. In contrast, Jakobson's use of the term "binary" referred to the abstracted feature itself, the *principium divisionis,* as he called it. The relationship between bilateral and binary therefore cannot be considered completely isomorphic. For example, the opposition /p/-/t/ or /b/-/d/ would be considered binary in the Jakobsonian classification, based on the abstracted feature contrast grave/acute. Within the Trubetzkoyan classification, on the other hand, the same oppositions /p/-/t/ and /b/-/d/ would have to be considered multilateral because the common core of these two phonemes, or the features shared between them, were also found in /k/. The oppositions between /p/-/b/, /t/-/d/, and /k/-/g/, on the other hand, would be considered binary by Jakobson and bilateral by Trubetzkoy as well, since the common core of each of these opposition pairs is not repeated in any other phoneme.

The difference between binary and bilateral therefore must be sought in the somewhat different base of the respective classifications of opposition relationships. For Trubetzkoy such a basis consisted of the common core of an opposition, and for Jakobson it consisted of an isolated feature. For Jakobson, binarity also extends to all features. This was not the case for the Trubetzkoyan concept of bilaterality. Only a limited number of oppositions were bilateral. In Jakobson's classification binary refers to both feature and opposition. For Trubetzkoy, bilateral can refer only to opposition. In developing his feature concept Jakobson was able, as will be seen, to break through the traditional points of articulation parameter and replace it by a series of new binary relations.[35] Trubetzkoy, though, was not able to do so. The points of articulation parameter was mirrored in the *heterogeneous* relationships in the above classification that Trubetzkoy found impenetrable. Jakobson's binarity thus extended to the entire phonological system, while the Trubetzkoyan bilaterality did not and could not because of the limitations of its framework.

In addition to the above difference, a further important fact added to differences in the scope of application of the two terms "binarity" and "bilaterality." Bilateral oppositions for Trubetzkoy also included gradual oppositions, which were oppositions in which the differential feature itself could be thought of as having more than two values. An example is the familiar aperture opposition, i-e-o. In the Trubetzkoyan system, the opposition of aperture was considered gradual, though bilateral. In the Jakobsonian classification gradualness and binarity are mutually exclusive.

One might ask whether the distinction between multilateral oppositions and gradual oppositions was really justified.

The difference between bilateral and multilateral oppositions hypothetically can be thought of in terms of the existence of an archiphoneme. In the case of bilateral oppositions, the archiphoneme has all the features the phonemes have in common, minus one + value of a feature. This is also true for the gradual oppositions (where the differential feature can be thought of as having three values, on a linear scale). In the case of multilateral oppositions, the number of features shared by the opposition members is fewer than for bilateral oppositions. Furthermore, the actual contrast is between no more than *two phonemes*. But also inherent in the classification into the multilateral category is the knowledge of what other phonemes occur in the rest of the system, since the classification is based on the analysis of the entire system. In the case of the gradual oppositions, the actual contrast is between *more than two phonemes*.

However, this circumstance alone is not sufficient to explain why some oppositions are considered gradual and others multilateral. For example, Trubetzkoy always considered the parameter of vocalic aperture as a (potential) gradual opposition. Jakobson analyzed vocalic aperture into two oppositions (compactness/noncompactness and diffuseness/nondiffuseness). This distinction had been originally introduced by Morris Halle in his 1957 exposition, *In Defense of the Number Two.* (For a discussion, see text p. 86.) In contrast, Trubetzkoy considered the point of articulation parameter multilateral. (It would be possible to think of this parameter as gradual, having one differential feature, that of "point of articulation.") Again, Jakobson analyzed this parameter further to include two oppositions, compactness and acuteness. Jakobson thus clearly demonstrated that both of these parameters, aperture and point of articulation, could be equally broken down further.

An explanation for the Trubetzkoyan distinction between gradual and multilateral oppositions might, perhaps, be thought in terms of psychological reality. It may be that for Trubetzkoy the aperture feature was more psychologically real as one feature and thus justified classification as a gradual opposition. The "point of articulation" parameter may have a different psychological reality. It also deserves mention that in the phonetic literature points of articulation have always been distinguished by individual labels. Other, secondary, differentiations along this parameter frequently also have been contingent on these primary labels. An example is the primary label "labial" and the secondary classification "labiodental," "bilabial," etc.

The concept of gradual opposition was part of a further distinction Trubetzkoy introduced into his bilateral category. Based on logical relations existing between two opposition members, he divided bilateral oppositions into privative, equipollent, and gradual oppositions. These were distinguished as follows:

Privative oppositions were oppositions in which one member had a feature the other member did not have. An example is the distinction between oral and nasal vowels in French, where the nasal vowels have the feature +nasal, which is absent in the oral vowels. *Equipollent oppositions* were those in which each member was characterized by a specific contrast feature. The same contrast features were always in the same opposition with each other. An example is the opposition strident/mellow, in which stridency is one contrast feature and mellow the other. *Gradual oppositions* were those whose members possessed different degrees of the same property. An example is the degree of aperture in vowels. Figure 2 extends this additional classification to the diagram in Figure 1 (p. 53).

Convertibility of Oppositions, Binarity, and Feature Hierarchy

The distinction between the three types of oppositions, privative, gradual, and equipollent, was not seen as absolute. How an opposition was interpreted in actual practice depended "more or less on the point of view from which one started" (Trubetzkoy, 1936c; p. 14) For example, the contrast between voiced and voiceless stops could be considered equipollent, that is, as having two contrastive features: the contrastive feature for /d/b/g/ would be the vibration of the vocal cords, which is absent in the voiceless stops. The contrast feature for /p/t/k/ would be the tensing of the buccal muscles, which is absent in voiced stops. The opposition between voiced and voiceless stops can also be considered privative. It becomes privative when only one of the features, vibration of the

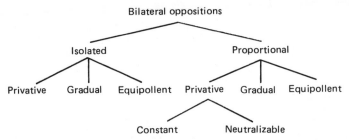

Figure 2. Extending the bilateral oppositions into the new classifications of privative, gradual, and equipollent.

vocal cords or tensing of the buccal musculature, is abstracted and considered distinctive. Trubetzkoy outlined guidelines to convert this type of opposition:

> . . . to interpret (these) relations as privative, attention must be focused on one property, and the lesser degree thereof must be equated with zero. (1939/1969, p. 76)

Gradual oppositions were also convertible into privative oppositions. For example, the opposition between long and short vowels in German could be considered gradual because degrees of vowel length were involved. But when length in the short vowels was considered a minimum, the relationship became privative, "since then the long vowels possessed the feature of exceeding the minimum in duration which is absent in the short vowels" (1936c, p. 15).

Conversely, privative oppositions were convertible into gradual oppositions. For example, the opposition between German "u" and "o" could be considered privative, that is, as open versus not open or closed versus not closed. Trubetzkoy maintained that in those cases where the same system also contained still another more open vowel, the open–not open contrast changed to a gradual relationship, e.g., u-o-a.

Gradual oppositions were also convertible to equipollent oppositions, as were equipollent oppositions into gradual ones. For example, the distinction between /s/ and /š/ in German was considered equipollent by Trubetzkoy. But if a language also contained a retroflex /ṣ/ the opposition changed to a gradual one.

Trubetzkoy's reference to a point of view from which one started and which appeared to play a role in assigning a contrast to one of these three opposition types, at least partially involved a distinction between a phonetic and a phonological level. He came close to spelling this out in *Grundzüge* when he said:

> A phonic opposition taken out of the context of the phonemic system and its functioning, and considered in isolation, is always at once equipollent and gradual. . . . whether an opposition must actually be considered as privative, gradual, or equipollent, depends on the structure and the functioning of the respective phonemic system. (1939/1969, p. 75)

Definitive judgments could thus only be made in the total context of a given system. The capacity to change from one category to another, at least in part, also appeared to reflect a difference between language-general or language-universal statements and language-specific statements. The three types of opposition represented phonological differences that Trubetzkoy uncovered in the course of his typological studies. He classed them one way on the basis of many similar phonological systems which he had analyzed. He classed them another based on the structure of the individual language under study. An example is his classification of sibilants as equipollent or gradual depending on whether a system contains two or three sibilants. For example, if the system contained /s/-/š/ the opposition was considered equipollent; if it contained /s/-/ṣ/-/š/ the opposition was considered gradual.

Thus, after Trubetzkoy had abstracted the three categories he did not consider assignment of a contrast to any one of them as absolute. It was possible to change within these categories. However, a final choice was not arbitrarily made in the classification of phonological oppositions. The choice depended on the phonological system of a given language. The possibility to convert from one to another category was thus really more rigidly controlled as would appear at first glance, both in cases where such changes occurred as well as on language-general grounds.

The distinction between the three opposition types, gradual, equipollent, and privative, actually appeared to exist on three levels, the phonetic level, a phonological (language-specific) level, and a typological (language-general) level.

Of the three types of oppositions, Trubetzkoy considered the privative oppositions the most important. This was true especially where such a contrast was supported by neutralization. In actual practice, however, the status of an opposition was determined by the phonological structure of the entire system of a given language. Consequently, Trubetzkoy was unable to convert all oppositions into binary and especially privative oppositions within his theoretical framework. Within his classification, he noted that the equipollent oppositions were the most numerous. He considered the feature status of their two members as "logically equivalent." Equipollent were those oppositions that were regarded neither as two degrees of one feature (gradual) nor as the absence or presence of a feature (privative).

The realization that opposition categories could be changed prompted Trubetzkoy in *Grundzüge* (1939/1969, p. 77) to modify the classification he had developed earlier in *Essai d'une theorie* (1936c). He now distinguished between those oppositions which were *logically* and those which were *actually* equipollent, gradual, and privative. The following diagram, replicated from *Grundzüge* (1939/1969, p. 77) indicates the extent to which Trubetzkoy found the three categories changeable from one to the other:

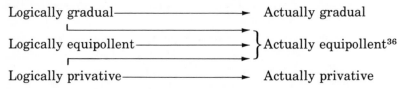

Logically gradual ⟶ Actually gradual

Logically equipollent ⟶ } Actually equipollent[36]

Logically privative ⟶ Actually privative

When oppositions were first categorized into correlations and disjunctions, the focus was on the presence versus the absence of a feature or property (cf. the definition of correlation, p. 3). Within the new framework, the earlier correlation was replaced by the category of proportional, privative oppositions. In the earlier framework, all other relationships had been subsumed under the term "disjunction." It is interesting to note that already in the earlier framework a certain amount of convertability existed between the disjunctions and the correlations, at least for Trubetzkoy. The following example illustrates this. In discussing the oppositions of localization *(Lokalisierungsgegensätze)*, that is, the oppositions based on point of articulation, Trubetzkoy made the following comment on the correlative/disjunctive classification:

> Acoustically speaking, every sound in these oppositions is contrasted with all other sounds. Consequently the oppositions must be considered as disjunctive. However, from an articulatory point of view, it is possible to convert these disjunctive oppositions into a number of correlative oppositions. (1931a, p. 103)

Thus, for example:

Glottal—v.—Oral
/   \
Lip—v.—Tongue
/   \
Dorsum—v.—Tip of tongue

Trubetzkoy nevertheless maintained that for phonology an acoustic viewpoint was more important. Accordingly, the oppositions had to remain disjunctive. An example is the oppositions created by the phonemes /p/-/t/ and /k/.

On the other hand, oppositions based on manner of articulation *(Artikulationsartgegensätze),* such as voiced/voiceless and, aspirated/unaspirated, always had to be considered correlative. If for some reason this was not possible, they had to be shifted to another type of opposition. This point can be illustrated by the opposition between spirants and occlusives, called *Annäherungskorrelation,*[37] translatable as "correlation of approximation." In *Grundzüge* it was also rendered as "correlation of occlusiveness or constriction." In *Die phonologischen System* Trubetzkoy said:

> However, it should be noted that the latter type of opposition here mentioned is not always correlative. In those instances where it is felt as disjunctive, it cannot be considered an opposition based on manner of articulation. It must be considered an opposition of localization. That is to say, occlusives and spirants are then conceived of as two different positions of the articulating organs and not as two degrees of mutual approximation of these organs. (1931a, p. 103)

The classification into correlations and disjunctions thus seemed to be rather inflexible in the case of manner of articulation. Instead of changing the classification to disjunctive, the opposition itself had to be shifted to another category.

A comparison of the Trubetzkoyan classification of oppositions with that of Jakobson immediately discloses that Jakobson by no means shared all the distinctions made by Trubetzkoy.

The Trubetzkoyan approach had essentially two foundations. First, oppositions were classified based on their relation to the entire system. This principle governed the bilateral/multilateral dichotomy. Second, oppositions were classified according to the relation of opposition members to each other. These two classificatory principles were, of course, interrelated. This is evident from the fact that bilateral oppositions were the ones on which the second type of classification was focused.

Jakobson, who had originally introduced the notion of correlation into phonology, also soon found that the initial classification into correlations and disjunctions was inadequate and that it obscured a great many relationships. He therefore abandoned it. However, unlike Trubetzkoy, he did not replace the earlier dichotomy by a more complex classification based on both the relationships between opposition members and the relationship between an opposition and the entire system. Instead, he seemed to concentrate on the type of information provided by the old correlations. That is to say, Jakobson concentrated on the relations among the opposition members themselves. By definition, these old correlations had been proportional in terms of the Trubetzkoyan classificatory system. This fact seems to have been helpful to Jakobson in abstracting the *principium divisionis* or division element that subsequently was to become the autonomous binary feature.

It is of interest to follow the fate of the type of information coded by the Trubetzkoyan classification based on the relationship of the individual opposition to the entire phonological system and to see how it remained relevant in the subsequent Jakobsonian classification. Initially, such information was simply lost within the framework of that classification.[38] However, belated concern for the pertinence of this type of information has appeared in recent questions bearing for example, on feature hierarchy. Distinctions such as isolated and proportional relations between features are found in generally unformalized shape. If feature diagrams and trees are studied carefully, this information becomes available in the number of existing pluses and minuses, the node at which a particular feature branches off in a tree, and the place in which a particular feature appears in the order of features in a chart (based on a +/− economy). The dichotomy between the Trubetzkoyan homogeneous and heterogeneous oppositions becomes relevant, for example, in determining whether or not a specific sequence of features has a fixed place in a hierarchy.[39]

A basic difference in the approaches of Trubetzkoy and Jakobson was that by reducing all oppositions to binary ones, Jakobson introduced a greater degree of simplicity, consistency, and abstraction into his analysis of phonological data, although by so doing he obscured some important information. In contrast, Trubetzkoy adhered more closely to phonetic reality which led to a more complex system of oppositions, yet at the expense of theoretical elegance.

Specific differences between the Trubetzkoyan and the Jakobsonian approaches lay in the types of oppositions they recognized. Where Trubetzkoy had recognized two types of contrast within his bilateral oppositions, namely, binary (privative and equipollent) and gradual oppositions, Jakobson only recognized one type, namely, binary oppositions.

Also within the Jakobsonian binary classification, the distinction between privative and equipollent oppositions appears to

have been lost, at least on the surface. Only privative oppositions remained. However, the distinction between privative and
equipollent oppositions had not always been absent from Jakobson's classification. Its loss represented a rather late development. The distinction was very much present in Jakobson's
Zur Struktur des Phonems (1939c), which represented his beliefs
at that time. Even in *Preliminaries to Speech Analysis* (1952),
co-authored by Fant and Halle, the following statement can still
be found:

> The listener is obliged to choose either between *two polar qualities* of
> the same category . . . or between *the presence and the absence of a
> certain quality.* (p.3; emphasis added).

However, in Jakobson's subsequent *Retrospect* (1962b), is this
statement:

> There are (privative) oppositions in which the absence of a property
> is *supplemented* by the presence of a contrary property. (emphasis
> added)

Jakobson thus appeared to have recognized the category of
equipollent oppositions, but very much in the disguise of privative oppositions. It may very well be possible that the attempt to
accommodate the equipollent oppositions within the privative
category was made in order to create a uniform framework for a
+/− notation.[40] A more important difference between the
Trubetzkoyan and Jakobsonian classification was the distinction
between gradual and binary oppositions. Where Trubetzkoy
recognized both gradual and binary oppositions, Jakobson recognized only binary ones. Jakobson was convinced of his binarity
principle early in his career. In *Zur Struktur des Phonems* he
noted: "The oppositions of distinctive properties are truly logical
binary oppositions"[41] (1939c/1962, p. 303). Even today Jakobson
cannot be shaken in his conviction that all oppositions, that is,
all features, are binary. The question of binarity versus nonbinarity has, of course, been an interesting and fruitful topic
for quite some time. Generative phonologists had hoped to have
settled it, at least within the context of their theory, by assigning
binary status to all features in a classificatory matrix, and
n-ary status to the features in a phonetic matrix. (Cf. above,
p. 18 ff.) For Jakobson:

> . . . the dichotomous scale is the pivotal principle of linguistic
> structure. The code imposes it upon the sound. (Jakobson, Fant,
> and Halle, 1952, p. 9)

Jakobson believed that this dichotomous principle was inherent in linguistic structure, where it was also supported by the principles of economy and simplicity, which have proved to be important evaluative criteria in linguistic descriptions. In his more recent work, Jakobson took a further step affirming his binarity principle when he theorized that the dichotomous scale may very well be built into the human central nervous system itself. For example, in *The Role of Phonic Elements in Speech Perception* (1966), Jakobson stated:

> A polarization method used by the nervous system changes our percepts into concepts. (p. 13)

Though such a claim is very challenging, it remains without proof.

Trubetzkoy concurred with Jakobson that from an abstract point of view it was possible to consider all oppositions as binary. However, ultimately Trubetzkoy's arguments were language specific. In the final analysis it was the structure and the function of a given phonemic system which were decisive in determining the privative, equipollent, or gradual nature of an opposition. The difference between the Trubetzkoyan and the Jakobsonian viewpoints with respect to binarity thus was twofold. First, whereas Jakobson only recognized binary relations, Trubetzkoy also recognized gradual relations. Second, for Jakobson, a language-specific feature system presented a selection from a universal set of binary features. In contrast, the distinction between typological (universal) and language-specific considerations in itself may have altered the status of an opposition from binary to gradual, or vice versa, in the Trubetzkoyan classification.

It is clear that without the Jakobsonian breakthrough in the classification of consonants, a consistent binary analysis would not have been possible. This breakthrough occurred in his 1938 exposition, *Observations sur le classement phonologique des consonnes*. Much later, the Jakobsonian binarity principle was attacked on grounds which appeared to have totally lost sight of the origins of that principle. Postal, in *Aspects of Phonological Theory* (1968), accused Jakobson of confusing two types of features:

> . . . phonetic features whose values are not exclusively binary, which are primitives of a system for describing ideal pronunciation, and systematic features, the binary projection of the right set of phonetic features which are relevant for the description of the phonological structure. . . . The difficulties are, of course, further compounded by

Jakobson's assumption that the binary features define autonomous phonemes rather than systematic features. (p. 110)

Seen in the light of historical developments in phonology, these comments are like putting the cart before the horse. Postal's criticism with respect to the first part was, of course, mistaken, and his comments with respect to the second part were correct but unfair. As has been shown, the distinctive feature concept developed out of the systematic breakdown of the phoneme. The phoneme had been considered a primitive before the distinctive feature itself became autonomous and was used independently. At the time the phoneme was defined as a bundle of distinctive features (1932; cf. p. 12) no such distinction as between autonomous and systematic phonemes had as yet been made. In fact, the very definition of the phoneme in the above terms constituted a landmark in phonology, a field which was not well established at that time. As to confusing phonetic and systematic features, it must be emphasized that from the very start the distinctive feature had been a relational abstract unit of the message code in the sense that the members of a distinctive opposition were never meant to be identical with any one phonetic value, but rather that the relation between the opposition members be the same. The distinction between "phonetic" and "systematic" values had clearly been recognized, as a statement by Trubetzkoy attests:

> Instrumental phonetics teaches that consonants are only rarely absolutely voiced or absolutely voiceless, most cases merely involve various degrees of voice participation. (1939/1969, p. 75)

The distinctive opposition voiced/voiceless therefore already clearly represented a binary abstraction from the phonetic level. Fant, in *The Nature of Distinctive Features* (1967), aptly expressed the relation of phonetics to the distinctive features:

> It is, of course, required that the physical and physiological manifestation be consistent, i.e., one and the same feature shall have *qualitatively* the same articulatory, acoustic, and perceptual correlates independent of context of other features within the bundle. The modification *"qualitatively"* here implies *that the relation between the two opposites is the same* in all contexts. (p. 635; emphasis added)

Fant was quick to underscore that:

> *Absolute values* of descriptive parameters, however, generally *vary with context*. Failure to recognize the role of contextual bias is a frequent source of misunderstanding of the nature of distinctive features. A distinctive feature is by definition the same in all con-

texts. The underlying physical phenomena, on the other hand, referred to as "correlates", "cues", or "parameters," need exhibit only *relational invariance*. (p. 635; emphasis added)

And:

Distinctive features are really distinctive categories or classes within a linguistic system, but just like in accepted phonemic analysis, it is required that they are consistent with the phonetic facts and these phonetic facts on various levels have lent their name to the features. (p. 635)

Jakobson (personal communication) claimed that Trubetzkoy was on the verge of being convinced of a consistent theory of binarity at the time he wrote *Grundzüge*. Unfortunately, time ran out on Trubetzkoy and we will never know just how far he agreed with Jakobson on the matter. It is clear, however, that Trubetzkoy was familiar with Jakobson's classification. For example, he adopted the strident/mellow dichotomy in *Grundzüge*. Strident/mellow had been an innovation in Jakobson's *Observations sur le classement phonologique des consonnes* (1938). Despite his familiarity with Jakobson's classification, however, Trubetzkoy continued to maintain the distinction between gradual, privative, and equipollent oppositions and their "logical" and "actual" variants in his final work, *Grundzüge*.

It is noteworthy that Trubetzkoy, unlike Jakobson, came back to the use of the concept of correlation in the framework of his new classification. However, the content of this concept was slightly altered.[42] As mentioned earlier, Trubetzkoy discarded the old concept of correlation in *Essai d'une théorie* (1936c). Fundamentally, the concept of correlation had captured an important and useful type of generalization about oppositive relationships. This apparently was not forgotten by Trubetzkoy and must account for his rediscovery of the notion in *Grundzüge*. There correlation derives its interpretation from the definitions of correlation pair and correlation mark.[43] A correlation, in this new classification, was the *sum of all correlation pairs* characterized by the same correlation mark. Put differently, correlations consisted of *logically* privative, proportional, bilateral oppositions which included several phoneme pairs.

In Trubetzkoy's new classification, the change in content compared to the earlier version of correlation thus was twofold. First, to qualify as a correlation an opposition now did not need to *actually* be privative—it only needed *to be conceived of* as privative. Second, a correlation now included the sum of all correlation pairs. Perhaps this point represents a small refinement over the earlier opposition series (*série d'oppositions;* cf. p. 3 ff.).

Trubetzkoy viewed those oppositions, which could also be considered correlations, as the most revealing of all opposition relationships. Accordingly, correlations in the above sense constituted a major unit of classification in *Grundzüge.*

In a comparison of the Trubetzkoyan and Jakobsonian feature system, the new Trubetzkoyan correlations assumed importance for two reasons. First, the distinction between gradual, equipollent, and privative oppositions became largely irrelevant on the level of correlations: as long as oppositions were bilateral, they could also be conceived of as *logically privative.* The relations between features were logical for Jakobson as well. In *On the Identification of Phonemic Entities* (1949/1962, p. 420) Jakobson noted: "The dichotomy of distinctive features is in essence a logical operation." The second reason for the importance of the correlation was that, because of the proportional character of the correlation, the feature involved became more visible and thus could be abstracted more easily and used independently. Jakobson did this when he shifted emphasis from opposition to feature in his later work.

Clearly, by the use of the concept of correlation[44] in its new form as "logically privative" Trubetzkoy was theoretically prepared to close the gap between his final classification and that of Jakobson in terms of binarity. Disagreement between the two then related mainly to the language-specific level, where the logically privative oppositions which could be interpreted as language general or language universal would have to be changeable to actually privative oppositions.

The fact, of course, remains that Trubetzkoy did not adopt the Jakobsonian binary consonant classification in his *Grundzüge.*

At this point it would be reasonable to ask whether the distinction between Trubetzkoy and Jakobson with respect to binarity could not be placed into a broader framework reflective of the spirit of the times. One may speculate, for example, that Jakobson may have been influenced by philosophical trends in thinking associated with phenomenology, which developed in Europe after the turn of the century under the impetus of Edmund Husserl and his *Logische Untersuchungen* (1928). Phenomenology may have provided the *Zeitgeist* for the development of the concept of logical relations in phonology and to an a priori conception of language universals. Jakobson repeatedly referred to Husserl and phenomenology in the course of his work (cf. *Retrospect,* 1962b). The distinction between logical and actual opposition relationships found in the work of Trubetzkoy may be interpreted as an attempt to accommodate two influences, that provided by Husserl and his phenomenology and that of Trubetzkoy's psychologist and psychologist-turned-linguist friend, Karl Bühler. Bühler repeatedly underscored the importance of evidence from concrete linguistic data for theoretical postulations and advocated a more "a posteriori" conception of linguistic structures. But even though some support for Jakobson's binarity principle could be sought in the influence of phenomenology, Jakobson, at the time he wrote *Observations sur le classement des consonnes* (1938), did not as yet put a premium on binarity. The preoccupation with an all inclusive binarity principle in Jakobson's later work perhaps may be seen as a parallel to the development of information theory and computer sciences in the United States from the late 1940s onward.[45]

EXPLORATION OF A BINARY
DISTINCTIVE FEATURE SYSTEM

After the preceding theoretical discussion, the actual development of a binary feature classification can now be examined. The following articles are the most relevant in the early development of a binary feature theory. They consist of Trubetzkoy's classification of vowel systems, *Zur allgemeinen Theorie der phonologischen Vokalsysteme* (1929a); his classification of vowels and consonants, in *Die phonologischen Systeme* (1931a); and Jakobson's classification of consonants, *Observations sur le classement phonologique des consonnes* (1938). After an examination of these initial contributions to binarity, the classificatory systems as they finally emerged are examined. These include Trubetzkoy, *Grundzüge der Phonologie* (1939/1969); Jakobson, Fant, and Halle, *Preliminaries to Speech Analysis* (1952); Jakobson and Halle, *Fundamentals of Language* (1956); and Chomsky and Halle, *The Sound Pattern of English* (1968).

The Chomsky-Halle classification of features differs from both that of Jakobson and that of Trubetzkoy. In some ways it comes closer to Trubetzkoy's classification. In order to explore some of the reasons for this particular direction of development, the relationship of the Chomsky-Halle classification to the earlier two classifications is also discussed.

Toward a Typology of Vowel Features

The first exhaustive classification of features was that given for vowels in Trubetzkoy's 1929 treatise, *Zur allgemeinen Theorie der phonologischen Vokalsysteme*.[46] According to this classification, every vowel phonetically consisted of a combination of several acts of articulation. Each vowel objectively had to have a specific degree of aperture (acoustically sonority), a specific position of articulation (acoustically timbre), a specific duration, expiratory force, and a specific tone movement.

However, for any one vowel only some of these features were distinctive. Trubetzkoy then set up a hierarchy of oppositions that also constituted a hierarchy of dependencies of oppositions (features) with respect to the vowels. What these were are discussed below.

Oppositions of Aperture or Sonority   These, Trubetzkoy maintained, were absolutely indispensable for any vowel system; they assumed primary status. Of the oppositions associated with the five acts of articulation listed above, it was possible that this one opposition alone was the one that is distinctive for a vowel system. Trubetzkoy cited the vowel system of Adyghe, a Caucasian language, as an example. He set up three vowel phonemes for this language: /ə/, which had a minimal degree of aperture; /e/, which had a mid degree of aperture; and /a/, which had a maximal degree of aperture.

Oppositions Based on Position of Articulation or Timbre   Trubetzkoy maintained that these oppositions (features) never occurred alone but only in conjunction with the oppositions of degree of aperture.[47] They related to a front-back classification (e.g., /i-e-u/).

With respect to the *opposition of duration* and *the opposition of expiratory force,* that is, stress or dynamic accent based on the acts of articulation listed above, Trubetzkoy maintained that only one of the them could be distinctive for one and the same language. Such a rule had been formulated originally by Jakobson in his 1923 *O česskom stiche*, and Trubetzkoy had incorporated it in his classification of vowels. Both German and English are considered exceptions to the above rule.

Trubetzkoy considered the oppositions of duration and stress as universal combinatory variants of *the opposition of intensity,* expressed in the one language by the opposition of long and short vowels, in the other by the opposition of stressed and unstressed vowels.

Both duration and expiratory force were considered vowel features. In the subsequent course of development in *Die phonologischen Systeme* (1931a) Trubetzkoy classed the two oppositions among the prosodic oppositions, however, still as a sub-classification of vocalic features. Still later, in *Grundzüge der Phonologie* (1939/1969), vocalic and prosodic features were ultimately established as two independent feature classes.

Jakobson also considered the prosodic features to be an independent class of features. In Jakobson and Halle (1956, p. 24 ff.) the following notations are found regarding the expiratory force and duration of quantity features:

> The observation of force and quantity in their intersyllabic variety seems to indicate that the prosodic distinctive features utilizing intensity and those utilizing quantity tend to merge.

And:

> Languages where both length and stress appear as distinctive are quite exceptional, and if the stress is distinctive, the latter is mostly supplemented by a redundant length.

The view taken in *Fundamentals* with respect to the relationship between expiratory force and duration thus is one of a general tendency rather than a universal law.

Based on these four oppositions, which phonetically were considered present in all vowels, Trubetzkoy set up four classes of vowel systems. These four classes related more specifically to the co-occurrence of oppositions as distinctive. They were:

Class I—Vowel systems in which only the aperture feature was distinctive

Class II—Vowel systems in which both aperture and timbre were distinctive

Class III—Vowel systems in which aperture, timbre, and intensity were distinctive

Class IV—Vowel systems in which aperture, timbre, intensity, and pitch were distinctive

Of these four distinctive features—aperture, timbre, intensity, and pitch—Trubetzkoy concluded that the aperture feature was primary. The aperture and the timbre features were the two basic correlates to any vowel system (except class I, which only had the aperture feature, but usually the timbre feature redundantly).

Differences among individual vowel systems were thus basically reducible to changes along either the vertical (aperture) or the horizontal (timbre) parameter. This meant that to determine the structure of any vowel system, it was important to determine how many degrees of aperture and classes of timbre could be distinguished phonologically. Any vowel system (except class IJ had to have at least two degrees of aperture and two classes of timbre. Based on these two oppositions, the opposition of aperture and the opposition of timbre (based on position of articulation), Trubetzkoy then set up two basic types of vowel systems into which, according to him, any vowel system could be classified. He called these *triangular* and *quadrangular*.

The essential difference between triangular and quadrangular systems consisted of the following: the triangular systems had only one phoneme of maximal degree of aperture and the opposition of timbre was nondistinctive for that phoneme. Trubetzkoy noted that such a phoneme was "outside of the classes of timbre." In contrast, the opposition of timbre was distinctive for all phonemes in the quadrangular systems, which had two phonemes of maximal degree of aperture. Figure 3 presents a tree diagram for these two systems.

Although these oppositions were basically binary in accordance with the above minimal systems, they were binary only in their minimal form. If a system contained more vowels, either along its horizontal or vertical axis, the oppositions became gradual. In accordance with the conditions of a given language, several degrees of aperture and several classes of timbre could be included in gradual oppositions. The gradual character of these oppositions therefore was not limited to ternary oppositions alone.

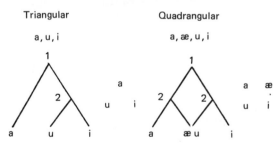

Figure 3. Tree diagram for Trubetzkoy's two systems, triangular and quadrangular. 1, open-close (aperture); 2, back-front (timbre).

That Trubetzkoy considered the oppositions of intensity and length in a somewhat different light is evident from the fact that he graphically represented these oppositions separately from his basic triangle and quadrangle. He represented them by supplemental triangles and quadrangles.

In summary, then, Trubetzkoy set up for the first time what he believed to be universal features for all vowel systems. From the point of view of language universals he considered these features binary, although they could assume a gradual character from a language-specific point of view. The basic oppositions for vowels in this early classification were the opposition of aperture (open/close) and the opposition of timbre (front/back). Secondary oppositions were the oppositions of intensity (duration) and of pitch or tone movement.[48]

Natural Feature Classes

The second article important in the development of distinctive features is Trubetzkoy's *Die phonologischen Systeme* (1931a). In contrast to his earlier *Zur allgemeinen Theorie der phonologischen Vokalsysteme, Die phonologischen Systeme* addressed itself to both vowels and consonants. Both these above articles were still written within the framework of correlations and disjunctions.

In *Die phonologischen Systeme* Trubetzkoy established an important concept in what he called "natural groupings" or "natural classes" (*Wesensverwandtschaftsgruppen*). Trubetzkoy coined the term based on his finding that not all phonological oppositions were related in the same way. His studies had shown that some oppositions had a closer affinity for each other than did others. Those oppositions, which were "felt to be more closely related and projected onto one plane on the basis of the speaker's linguistic consciousness," also needed to be classified into special natural classes[49] to indicate their affinity for each other. In *Die phonologischen Systeme* Trubetzkoy established three such natural classes for the vowels and four for the consonants. All oppositions which existed in a given language also had to belong to one such class. The natural classes for the vowels were the following three:

1. *Oppositions of quality:*
    Aperture (sonority)
    Timbre
        Rounding correlation
        Palatovelar correlation (front versus back)

2. *Oppositions of resonance:*
   Nasalized versus non-nasalized
   Squeezed versus pure vowels
   Pharyngeal versus nonpharyngeal sounds
3. *Prosodic Oppositions:*
   Intensity:
   Dynamic
   Accented versus unaccented
   Weak versus strong
   Quantity
   Long versus short
   Melody (pitch)
   Tone movement
   Register
   Oppositions of close contact

In comparison with the earlier vowel classification in *Zur allgemeinen Theorie,* this classification had undergone considerable expansion.[50] It is noteworthy that the earlier two basic oppositions, those of aperture and timbre, had now been classed together under one natural class, "oppositions of quality." Trubetzkoy now maintained that the opposition of aperture was not correlative (that is, binary) but disjunctive. He had not specifically claimed this in the earlier *Zur allgemeinen Theorie.* Disjunctiveness referred to the gradual character which the opposition of aperture could assume when the basic vowel triangle or quadrangle was extended to reflect the phonological character of a particular language. In contrast, the oppositions of timbre, which in *Zur allgemeinen Theorie* could clearly assume gradual character depending on the number of vowels present in a given language, were now broken down into two correlations. These were the rounding and the palatovelar (front/back) correlations. Neither of these had been mentioned specifically in *Zur allgemeinen Theorie,* where the opposition of timbre had simply covered the horizontal parameter. Accordingly, the potentially gradual character of the opposition of timbre was here resolved into two binary oppositions: rounded/unrounded and front/back.

The third type of oppositions subsumed under the major class of "oppositions of quality" is the opposition of tenseness (that is, tense/lax). This is a newly added opposition which had not been mentioned in *Zur allgemeinen Theorie.* The opposition of tension reduces, although not entirely, the potentially gradual character of the vertical parameter of aperture of *Zur allgemeinen Theorie.*[51]

The resonance category of oppositions had not been discussed at all in *Zur allgemeinen Theorie*. This newly established class comprised the opposition between nasalized and non-nasalized vowels.[52] Trubetzkoy formulated the following general rule governing the occurrence of nasalized and non-nasalized vowels (the rule was subsequently also incorporated into the list of linguistic universals[53]): in any given system nasalized vowels are always fewer than non-nasalized vowels.

The two oppositions between squeezed and pure vowels and between pharyngealized and nonpharyngealized vowels were subsequently referred to as the "correlation of muffling" (Trubetzkoy, 1939/1969, p. 121 ff.). The earlier distinction between pure and squeezed vowels and pharyngealized/nonpharyngealized vowels was dropped. Apparently Trubetzkoy considered himself on uncertain grounds and the source literature on the subject inadequate for definite statements.

The opposition of intensity was subdivided in *Die phonologischen Systeme* into the opposition of dynamic stress and the opposition of quantity. It was already present in *Zur allgemeinen Theorie,* as was the opposition of melody (pitch). All three of these oppositions were now grouped together under the major class of prosodic oppositions. However, the prosodic oppositions still belonged to the vowel classification.

The opposition of melody was now subdivided into the opposition of tone movement (*Tonverlaufsgegensätze*), for example, falling-rising pitch, and the opposition of tone register (*Tonelagegegensätze*), for example, high, level, and low register.

In addition, a third type of prosodic opposition was added. This was the opposition between open and close contact (*Silbenschnittgegensatz* or *Gipfelstellungsgegensatz*). This represented an opposition based on different positions of the syllable crest: in the case of vowels with close contact, it is supposed to coincide with the end of vowel articulation and the implosion of the following consonant. In the case of open contact it does not so coincide. Where this distinction was present, it was found that length was redundant.[54]

With respect to the consonants, four major (natural) classes were set up in *Die phonologischen Systeme*:

1. *Oppositions of localization* (oppositions based on point of articulation)

2. *Oppositions of manner of articulation:*
   Voice correlation
   Correlation based on type of expiration
      Aspirated/unaspirated
      Glottalized/nonglottalized
   Constriction correlation (see p. 61 regarding the shift of this opposition to a different category)
3. *Oppositions of timbre:*
   Palatalized/nonpalatalized
   Rounded/unrounded
   Emphatic palatalization/nonemphatic palatalization
   Emphatic velarization/nonemphatic velarization
   Retroflex/dental
4. *Oppositions of intensity:*
   Dynamic
      Fortis/lenis
      Squeezed/nonsqueezed (*gedrängt/locker*)
      Strong/weak
   Quantity
      Long/short
      Geminated/nongeminated

In some cases Trubetzkoy expressed uncertainty regarding the assignment to natural classes. First, he was not sure how to interpret the relationship between sonorants and obstruents, that is, between sonorants and occlusives and fricatives. The problem, as he saw it, was whether these should be assigned to oppositions based on manner of articulation (class 2, above), or whether they should make up a separate class of oppositions of resonance which had not been included as a class in the above classification.

The second problem was related to the classification of liquids. Although Trubetzkoy clearly recognized that these formed a natural class, the problem lay in the discovery of their true opposites. In the above classification of consonants, only the oppositions of localization were not seen as binary.

At the time Trubetzkoy wrote *Die phonologischen Systeme,* he considered the acoustic correlates to his classificatory scheme more relevant than the articulatory aspect. Thus, in regard to the oppositions of localization Trubetzkoy maintained that even though it was feasible to analyze the point of articulation parameter into a series of binary oppositions from an articulatory point of view, it was not possible to do so from an acoustic point of view (also see above p. 60 ff.). He wrote:

> Acoustically speaking each articulatory position can be viewed as having its own specific sound (noise). However, such a sound is not specifically opposed to any other sound. *Instead, it contrasts with all other specific sounds.* And since for phonology acoustic considerations are far more important than articulatory considerations, oppositions of localization always remain disjunctive phonologically.[55] (1931a, p. 103; emphasis added)

Nothing is said in *Die phonologischen Systeme* with respect to the possible relationship between natural classes which Trubetzkoy set up for the vowels and those set up for consonants. Neither is there any mention made about the commonality of properties of vowels and consonants, although the oppositions for vowels and consonants in many cases carry the same name. In this context, and based on the fact that a phonological system usually has more consonants than vowels, Trubetzkoy pointed out that it was natural for a classification of consonants to be more complex than a classification of vowels.

It is interesting to note that Trubetzkoy had already used the classification of vowels as outlined above in an earlier study, *Polabische Studien* (1929c), without discussing it in any detail; he merely mentioned it as a practical application.

Polabische Studien also contains—for the first time, as far as can be determined—a consistent binary breakdown of a vowel system consisting of more than three or four vowels. The vowel system of Polabian, according to Trubetzkoy, had eight short vowels. His analysis of them is shown in Table 3.

> Based on position of articulation, the short vowels could be divided into "front" vowels (acoustically having "clear timbre"—/e, i, ö, ü/) and "back" vowels (acoustically having "dark timbre"—/a, ə, o, u/) . . . Based on lip rounding, the "back" vowels in turn were divided into "unrounded" (/a, ə /), and "rounded" (/u, o/) vowels . . .) . . . accord-

Table 3.   Trubetzkoy's vowel system for Polabian

	Back (dark Timbre)		Front (clear timbre)	
	Rounded	Unrounded	Rounded	Unrounded
Open	o	a	ö	e
Close	u	ə	ü	i

From *Polabische Studien* (Trubetzkoy, 1929c, p. 129).

ingly the "front" vowels also were divided into "rounded" (/ö, ü/) and "unrounded" (/e, i/). Finally, all short vowels, based on their degree of aperture (or sonority) could be divided into "open" vowels (acoustically having a greater degree of sonority (/a, o, e, ö/) and "close" vowels (acoustically having a lesser degree of sonority (/ə, u, i, ü/). Thus the Polabian system of short vowels showed quite a symmetrical structure. (1929c, p. 129)

Figure 4 assembles this information into a tree diagram, which can be represented as follows: (1) front-back, (2) rounded-unrounded, (3) open-close: It may be assumed that the binarity shown in this figure was incidental and that symmetry was the noteworthy phenomenon for Trubetzkoy. It appears that the various types of opposition only became the subject of systematic analysis in the subsequent *Die phonologischen Systeme*.

The Binary Analysis of the Point of Articulation Parameter

The binary analysis of the point of articulation parameter constituted a major breakthrough in the systematic application of the binarity principle in feature analysis. It was accomplished in Jakobson's *Observations sur le classement phonologique des consonnes* (1938).

As noted earlier, Trubetzkoy's preceding two articles had been written in the framework of correlations and disjunctions, as had *Polabische Studien*. In *Observations* Jakobson took direct issue with the Trubetzkoyan classification of consonants in terms of oppositions of localization as they appeared in *Die phonologischen Systeme*. Trubetzkoy had reduced all phonological differences between consonants to binary oppositions, with one exception: oppositions based on point of articulation. As stated earlier,

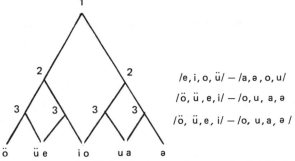

Figure 4. Tree diagram for Trubetzkoy's vowel system in *Polabische Studien*. 1, front-back; 2, rounded-unrounded; 3, open-close.

the classification also included some juggling between the parameters of manner and point of articulation (cf. above p. 59 ff.).

In *Die phonologischen Systeme* Trubetzkoy insisted that even though oppositions of localization could be considered binary (correlative) from an articulatory point of view, they could not be considered binary from an acoustic point of view. He persisted in his attitude of considering them disjunctive because, in his opinion, the acoustic aspects were more important than the articulatory aspects.

Jakobson could not agree more with Trubetzkoy's statement that "for phonology, acoustic considerations were far more important than articulatory considerations." So, for example, it is stated in *Preliminaries*:

> The closer we are in our investigation to the destination of the message (i.e., its perception by the receiver), the more accurately can we gage the information conveyed by its shape. This determines the operational hierarchy of levels of decreasing pertinence, perceptual, aural, acoustical, and articulatory (the latter carrying no direct information to the receiver).[56] (Jabokson, Fant, and Halle, 1952, p. .12)

However, Jakobson at the same time insisted that the description of any stage of the speech event must be convertible into any other stage:

> ... the specifications of the phonemic oppositions may be made in respect to any stage of the speech event from articulation to perception and decoding, on the sole condition that the variables of any antecedent stage be selected and correlated in terms of the subsequent stages ... (ibid., p. 13)

The limitations to binarity which Trubetzkoy had reached in *Die phonologischen Systeme* were ingeniously resolved by Jakobson in *Observations sur le classement des consonnes* (1938) by a change in parameters for the classification of consonants along the horizontal axis, that is, by a change in the previous point of articulation classification. Instead of classifying the consonants in terms of points of articulation, Jakobson found a common and differential denominator in the shape and volume of the oral resonance chambers. He then successfully combined these newly found articulatory parameters for the consonants with certain acoustic observations and thus established acoustic correlates for his newly found division as well.

Starting from the observation that in many languages a close relationship could be observed between velars and labials, Jakobson found that what these sounds had in common was their "long, undivided oral resonator" as opposed to the palatals and dentals, which had two small resonance chambers. Furthermore, in the production of the velars and labials the pharynx was retracted, but this retraction did not occur with the palatals and the dentals:

> Velars and labials take their specific character from a long, undivided oral resonator, while for the palatals and dentals the tongue divides the oral cavity into two short resonance chambers . . . the pharynx is retraced for velars and labials, while it is expanded for the corresponding palatals and dentals. (Jakobson, 1938/1962, p. 274)

Having grouped the velars and labials—as contrasted to the palatals and dentals—as grave versus acute consonants, Jakobson then further grouped velars and palatals (including sibilants) together, uniting them under the term "back consonants" (*postérieurs*) and opposing them to the labials and dentals, which he classed as "front consonants" (*antérieurs*). The specific feature separating the back from the front consonants was their point of articulation. For the back consonants the point of articulation was behind and for the front consonants it was in front of the only or dominant resonance chamber:

> Similarly, the velars and palatals, including the sibilants, are opposed to the labials and dentals by means of a specific characteristic. By grouping velars and palatals (including sibilants) under "back consonants" and labials and dentals under "front consonants" the following rule can be stated: for the back consonants the point of articulation is behind the only or major resonance chamber and for the front consonants it is in front of it. (1938/1962, p. 27)

Jakobson thus reduced the velars, palatals, dentals, and labials to two oppositions articulatorily, based on shape and volume of resonance chambers. Actually, it was not Jakobson who introduced this new parameter into phonology. It had already been present with respect to the vowels (cf. Trubetzkoy, *Zur allgemeinen Theorie*).[57] However, Jakobson did extend it to the consonants. Similarly, with respect to the opposition grave/acute, the terms "grave" and "acute" had already been in use for the vowels (cf. Jakobson, *Phonemic Notes on Standard Slovak*, 1931/1962, p. 221 ff.).

Jakobson then examined the above oppositions from an acoustic point of view and found that for the back consonants, as opposed to the front consonants, the distinction was one of higher degree of perceptibility, often accompanied by a greater degree of duration:

> . . . the back consonants are contrasted with the corresponding front consonants by means of a greater degree of perceptibility frequently accompanied, ceteris paribus, by a longer duration. (1938/1962, p. 274)

The distinction between the class of labials and velars (grave) on the one hand, and the class of dentals and palatals (acute) on the other, was that the former had a relatively dark timbre and the latter had a relatively clear timbre.

> A long and undivided resonator as well as a retracted back orifice lends a characteristic and relatively dark timbre to the velar and labial consonants. It corresponds to the timbre of the velar vowels and contrasts with that of the palatal and dental consonants. The timbre of the palatal and dental consonants is relatively clear and almost corresponds to the characteristic timbre of the palatal vowels. (1938/1962, p. 274)

What is here termed "acoustic" is not necessarily acoustic as it is used in *Preliminaries to Speech Analysis* and *Fundamentals of Language*. The term as used in *Observations* should be interpreted as "impressionistically" acoustic. In contrast, the term was used in the sense of "instrumentally" acoustic in *Preliminaries* and *Fundamentals*. But already in *Observations* Jakobson was attempting to relate this classification to acoustic experiments (cf. 1938/1962, p. 274).

In *Preliminaries* and *Fundamentals* the terms "back" and "front" consonants were replaced by the terms "compact" and "diffuse." The opposition was now described in instrumental-acoustic terms:

> . . . compact phonemes are characterized by the relative predominance of one centrally located formant region (or formant). They are opposed to diffuse phonemes in which one or more non-central formants or formant regions predominate. (Jakobson, Fant, and Halle, 1952, p. 27)

In *Fundamentals,* the distinction was acoustically refined:

> . . . higher (v. lower) concentration of energy in a relatively narrow, central region of the spectrum, accompanied by an increase (v. decrease) of the total amount of energy. (Jakobson and Halle, 1956, p. 29)

In *Preliminaries* the opposition compact/diffuse was differentiated in articulatory terms:

The essential articulatory difference between the compact and diffuse phonemes lies in the relation between the volume of the resonating cavities in front of the narrowest stricture and those behind this stricture. The ratio of the former to the latter is higher for the compact than for the corresponding diffuse phonemes. Hence the consonants articulated against the hard or soft palate (velars and palatals) are more compact than the consonants articulated in the front part of the mouth. (Jakobson, Fant, and Halle, 1952, p. 27)

In *Fundamentals* compact versus diffuse was differentiated in articulatory terms:

> ... forward-flanged versus backward-flanged. The difference lies in the relation between the volume of the resonance chamber in front of the narrowest stricture and behind this stricture. The ratio of the former to the latter is higher for the forward-flanged phonemes (wide vowels, and velar and palatal, including post-alveolar consonants) than for the corresponding backward-flanged phonemes (narrow vowels, and labial and dental, including alveolar consonants). (Jakobson and Halle, 1956, p. 29)

A similar change and sharpening of definitions can be seen with respect to the grave/acute dichotomy. In *Preliminaries* the opposition grave/acute was differentiated in instrumental-acoustic terms:

> Acoustically this feature means predominance of one side of the significant part of the spectrum over the other. When the lower side of the spectrum predominates, the phoneme is labeled grave; when the upper side predominates, we term the phoneme acute. (Jakobson, Fant, and Halle, 1952, p. 29)

In *Fundamentals* the acoustic correlate was given as:

> ... concentration of energy in the lower (vs. upper) frequencies of the spectrum. (Jakobson and Halle, 1956, p. 31)

In articulatory terms, the opposition was differentiated in *Preliminaries* in the following way:

> The gravity of a consonant or vowel is generated by a larger and less comparted mouth cavity, while acuteness originates in a smaller and more divided cavity. Hence gravity characterizes labial consonants as against dentals, as well as velars versus palatals. (Jakobson, Fant, and Halle, 1952, p. 30).

In *Fundamentals*, the articulatory distinction was given as:

> ... peripheral v. medial: peripheral phonemes (velar and labial) have an ampler and less compartmented resonator than the corresponding medial phonemes (palatal and dental). (Jakobson and Halle, 1956, p. 31)

A comparison of the first binary classification of the two oppositions discussed shows that Jakobson, after successfully applying the dichotomous scale in *Observations,* together with Halle
subsequently refined his articulatory specifications with a slight
shift in emphasis. However, what must be considered as much
more important is the replacement of impressionistic acoustic
corollaries, even though allusions were made to instrumental-
acoustic data, by a consistent effort at an instrumental-acoustic
classification in *Preliminaries* and *Fundamentals.*[58]

Observations, in addition to analyzing the previous point of
articulation parameter into two binary oppositions, was further
important in that Jakobson likened the acoustic impressions related to these consonantal oppositions to those found in the vowel
oppositions. Furthermore, he gave instances of the practical application for these features. For example, by using these features,
he was able to relate contextual changes in vowel or consonant to
a single feature. Thus, a segment which was +consonant, +grave
could change to +consonant, +acute in the environment of
+vocalic, +acute.

Whereas in Trubetzkoy's *Die phonologischen Systeme* (1931a)
the classificatory status of nasal versus oral consonants had not
yet been decided, in *Observations* Jakobson proposed to oppose
the nasals to the orals as follows:

> Nasal consonants as opposed to oral consonants are the result of a
> divided passage way. (1938/1962, p. 276)

Jakobson considered these three oppositions—grave/acute,
compact/diffuse, and oral/nasal, all based on a "different place
and structure of the resonators"—as the kernel of any phonological system. At the same time he called attention to their importance in first language acquisition:

> ... it is to these three consonant oppositions that some archaic types
> of primitive language and also child language are limited.[59] (1938/
> 1962, p. 276)

In *Observations* Jakobson pointed out further that all three of
these oppositions found their exact equivalent in the vowels. He
observed, however, that the compact consonants and vowels were
divided into grave/acute much more rarely than the diffuse consonants and vowels. He wrote:

The chasm found in earlier handbooks between the structure of consonants and that of vowels is justly challenged by modern acoustic science and seems to be bridged in the study of phonology. (ibid.)

Jakobson here pointed to the basic similarity between the consonant quadrangle and triangle constituted by the grave/acute and compact/diffuse dichotomies, and the vowel quadrangle and triangle which had been established earlier by Trubetzkoy (see earlier discussion, p. 71).

The liquids which Trubetzkoy had left unanalyzed vis-à-vis the phonological system were incorporated in *Observations* into the analysis of the feature system. Trubetzkoy had recognized the correlative relationship between the liquids. However, he was not sure how the liquids should be characterized vis-à-vis the entire system. Jakobson was able to distinguish the liquids from the rest of the consonants "by the simultaneous opening and closing of the buccal passage" (1938/1962, p. 278.) It seems that this definition of the liquids in *Observations* already pointed the way to their classification in terms of a split of the vocalic/consonantal features found in *Preliminaries* and *Fundamentals*. The split appears to have been caused, at least partially, by Jakobson's desire to accommodate the liquids into a unified system of distinctive features. In *Observations* the liquids had been opposed to each other in terms of the simultaneous closure of the oral cavity:

> ... *for the laterals* the two aforesaid simultaneous actions are in fact implemented at the same time, *but at two different places,* while for the trills *opening and closure occurs at the same place, but in succession.* (1938/1962, p. 278; emphasis added)

Jakobson established yet another binary opposition for the consonants in *Observations*: the opposition strident/mellow. As mentioned, in *Die phonologischen Systeme* Trubetzkoy shifted any opposition of constriction (*Annäherungsopposition*), when it was not binary (correlative), from the oppositions based on manner of articulation to the oppositions of localization (cf. above, p. 60). The oppositions based on manner of articulation were inherently binary for Trubetzkoy, while the oppositions of localization were not. Jakobson resolved this situation when he established the opposition strident/mellow. He thus accommodated the classification of the affricates (such as the oppositions t-t͡s and p-p͡f in German). In *Die phonologischen Systeme* Trubetzkoy grouped these under the opposition of constriction (stops/fricatives), an opposition which he considered gradual. (For the subsequent Trubetzkoyan framework for stridency in *Grundzüge*, refer to text discussion, p. 112 ff.).[61]

The stridents in *Observations* were characterized by:

> ... forceful turbulence caused by the expiring air resulting in a sharp tone.. An additional obstacle participating in this friction thus distinguishes the articulation of the strident fricatives from that of the mellow fricatives (1938/1962, p. 277)

The additional barrier or obstacle which related to stridency changed from one opposition pair to the next. For example, in the case of the opposition bilabial/labiodental, the bilabials only involved the lips, while the labiodentals also involved the (lower) teeth. With respect to the opposition of velars and uvulars, the soft palate and the back of the tongue were decisive for the velars, while the uvula was involved as well for the uvulars.

In addition to accommodating the affricate/stop distinction, the opposition strident/mellow thus allowed for further distinction within the compact/diffuse and grave/acute dichotomies.

In *Preliminaries* strident phonemes were primarily characterized:

> ... by a noise which is due to turbulence at the point of articulation. This strong turbulence in its turn, is a consequence *of a more complex impediment* which distinguishes the strident from the mellow consonants (Jakobson, Fant, and Halle, 1952, p. 2; emphasis added)

Acoustically, strident sounds are *"sounds that have irregular wave forms ... as opposed to mellow sounds that have regular wave forms"* (p. 23). In *Fundamentals* the distinction between strident and mellow sounds is presented as acoustically related to *"higher intensity noise versus lower intensity noise"* and genetically to *"rough-edged versus smooth-edged."*[62]

Jakobson in *Observations* left open the classification of both labiovelars and retroflexes. These were accommodated subsequently by Trubetzkoy in *Grundzüge* by the opposition flat/plain (cf. below, p. 117 ff.) and adopted by Jakobson into *Preliminaries* and *Fundamentals*.

Already in *Observations* Jakobson noted that the number of differential properties was much more restricted than the number of phonemes. Ivić, who reviewed Jakobson's contributions to phonology (1965), pointed out that the system of oppositions as it appeared in *Observations* was not yet the system of oppositions ultimately developed by Jakobson. In *Roman Jakobson and the*

Growth of Phonology (1965b, p. 61) Ivić noted that the system as it stood at the time of *Observations* still contained gradual oppositions for vowels (aperture). These had not yet been split. The glides also had not yet been accommodated. The relationship between /r/ and /l/ had not been interpreted in terms of the opposition interrupted versus continuant, and the features flat/nonflat, checked/unchecked, and sharp/plain had not yet been included. Ivić further called attention to the fact that the classificatory system at the time of *Observations* was still closer to immediately observable data. This meant that it was also less economical and less consistent in binary analysis.

Jakobson had not presented the entire system of oppositions. *In Observations,* he had merely taken issue with the nonbinary "point of articulation" parameter of Trubetzkoy's *Die phonologischen Systeme,* though generally crediting Trubetzkoy for developing a system of distinctive oppositions in binary terms.

Subsequent Fate of the Features
Grave/Acute and Compact/Diffuse

The oppositions grave/acute and, especially, compact/diffuse were established in *Observations* and have since been variously criticized and taken to task in the literature. Detailed criticism and sources of criticism can be found in Ivić (1965b, p. 57 ff.).

Much criticism has been directed to the accuracy of the details of their acoustic correlates (Romportl, 1963) and the relations of psychological space (Greenberg and Jenkins, 1964; Miller and Nicely, 1955). Experiments supported the existence of a close link between /k/-/t/ and /b/-/d/. However, experimental findings have also demonstrated more "psychological" distance between /k/ and /p/ and /g/ and /b/ than between /k/ and /t/ and /g/ and /d/. The former two pairs (/k/ and /p/ and /g/ and /b/ are linked by the feature of gravity. These findings have further shown that /k/ is confused more frequently with /θ/ and /s/ than with /š/, even though the feature compactness should bind /k/ more closely to /š/ than to /θ/ or /s/. The wisdom and reality of identifying the compact/diffuse division in consonants (horizontal parameter) with the aperture feature (vertical parameter) for the vowels has also been called into question (cf. Ivič, 1965b, p. 59 ff.).

Brozović (1967, p. 412 ff.) discussed the grave/acute and compact/acute and compact/diffuse features in terms of usefulness and maintained that diffuseness is less useful than compactness (/p,t/-/k,ć/) and that in regard to the opposition grave/acute, the high tonality of /t/ and /ĉ/ in turn is more useful than the low tonality of /p/ and /k/. Brozović pointed out further that even though the opposition compact/diffuse mirrored in /a/-/i,u/ is by far superior for the vowels, this is not true for the consonants, where the compact/diffuse opposition results in contrasting /k/ to /p,t/. He maintained that for the consonants contrasting /p/ to /k,t/ would be superior from a practical point of view.

With the inclusion of the vowels into the compact/diffuse dichotomy, the ± notation for the mid open vowel also belied true binarity. Even after the split of the compact/diffuse feature into compact/noncompact and diffuse/nondiffuse (cf. Halle, 1957), the binary principle was violated, although binarity was observed on the surface. The feature split there had to be considered a bit of hocus-pocus to achieve symmetry in the system rather than to reflect the reality of the phonological system.

The criticism of the above oppositions compact/diffuse and grave/acute subsequently became suspended in the light of a revised feature approach to what Chomsky and Halle have now termed "primary cavity features." The feature revision was in response to both criticism and inadequacies of the former classification (cf. also McCawley, 1967).

Chomsky and Halle wrote in *The Sound Pattern of English:*

> This complete identification of vowel and consonant features [in terms of gravity, compactness, and diffuseness] seems in retrospect to have been too radical a solution . . . We have therefore made a number of changes in the framework, in particular, with regard to the primary cavity features. The revised framework is quite likely to appear to depart from the earlier framework much more rapidly than it in fact does. (1968, p. 303)

Chomsky and Halle continue that:

> This deceptive impression is the result of the unfortunate need to change terminology once again and to replace the by now reasonably familiar terms compact, diffuse, and grave in part by totally new terms that are *a return to the status ante quo.* (1968, p. 303; emphasis added)

Chomsky and Halle (1968) described only the articulatory correlates of their features. Their reason for doing so was not because other aspects (acoustic and the perceptual) "are less interesting or less important, but rather . . . because it would make the book too long." It is clear that such an attitude must leave any criticism with respect to the acoustic correlates of compactness and gravity unanswered and in abeyance.[63]

In the Chomsky-Halle feature classification of *The Sound Pattern of English,* the shape and volume of the resonator cavity used by Jakobson as a base for feature differentiation was replaced by a new parameter. Feature differentiation became based on and related to the body of the tongue and the location of the obstruction in the oral cavity. The point of reference for the tongue was its position in its neutral state. However, neutral state of the tongue did not mean its position in its relaxed state, at the floor of the mouth. Chomsky and Halle understood neutral state of tongue to mean raised "to about the level that it occupies in the articulation of the English vowel /e/." According to them, their new classification did away with earlier differences between the physical correlates to vowels and consonants for the oppositions compact/diffuse and grave/acute which had existed in the Jakobsonian classification.

The oppositions compact/diffuse and grave/acute in the Chomsky-Halle classification were partly replaced by the opposition coronal/noncoronal, and anterior/nonanterior. However, they are not entirely identical. These two new Chomsky-Halle features are supplemented by the features high, low, and back. Table 4 shows the new Chomsky-Halle feature classification as it relates to the English phonological system, compared to the earlier Jakobsonian features as they relate to the phonological features of English.

Chomsky and Halle also established the features high/nonhigh, low/nonlow, and back/nonback. All of these are related to the placement of the body of the tongue as well. For the feature high, the tongue is raised to a level above its neutral position; for the feature low, it is lowered below its neutral position; and for the feature back, it is retracted from its neutral position. All five features are used for consonants and vowels. It deserves pointing out, however, that Chomsky and Halle did not succeed in establishing a fully symmetrical system. A relative asymmetry existed between the vowels and the consonants. Vowels were always noncoronal and nonanterior. The presence of the features +vocalic, −consonantal thus always made the specification noncoronal and nonanterior redundant.[64]

The Fate of the Stridency Feature

The existence of the stridency feature, which had also been established by Jakobson in *Observations,* subsequently was also challenged. Harris, in *Sound Change in Spanish and the Theory of*

Table 4. Chomsky-Halle classification (coronal/noncoronal and anterior/nonanterior) and correspondences in the Jakobsonian classification

Chomsky-Halle classification	Articulatory correlates	Correspondences in Jakobsonian classification
Coronal Alveolars, dentals, palatoalveolars, liquids produced with the blade of the tongue, retroflexes	Blade of tongue raised from neutral position	Acute—all of these, except palatal sounds, and addition of retroflexes
Noncoronal Labials, palatals, uvular R, vowels, glides y and w	Sounds not produced with the blade of the tongue (lip articulation, body of tongue)	Grave—in part, except that body of tongue also includes palatals, which are acute
Anterior Labials, dentals, alveolars, (front) liquids	Obstruction located in front of palatoalveolar region of mouth	Diffuse
Nonanterior Vowels, palatoalveolars, retroflexes, palatals, velars, uvulars, pharyngeals	Obstruction not located in front of palatoalveolar region of mouth	Compact, some flat

Marking (1969), claimed that stridency appeared to be a redundant feature:

> It must be asked at this point whether the feature [strident] really exists at all, that is, whether there are any two segments which differ *only* in stridency, and whether there are any rules in which [strident] cannot be eliminated without loss of generality. These questions must obviously remain open at present, but some preliminary investigation suggests that [strident] is entirely redundant. (p. 547)

Harris, of course, could not have made this statement within the framework of the Jakobsonian distinctive features. His observations are contingent and a result of the feature reclassification into *coronal, anterior, high, low,* and *back,* and the addition of the features *distributed* and *delayed release* in the Chomsky-Halle framework. (The above is representative of the fact that features and feature systems have an internal structure. A change in some part of this structure has as a consequence a change in the other parts of the same system.)

The feature *stridency* was still included in the Chomsky-Halle framework of *The Sound Pattern of English,* but its application was restricted (also see below, p. 113).

The feature *distributed* as represented in *The Sound Pattern of English* was, among other things, to provide for differentiation in the prepalatal region in cases where more than three points of articulation were present. An example of a language where this is the case is Toda, a language of India, which reportedly has five stops in the prepalatal region, /p, t̪, t, ʈ, k/: labial, dental, alveolar, retroflex, and palatoalveolar, respectively.

Distributed sounds are opposed to nondistributed sounds as sounds:

> ... with a constriction that extends for a considerable distance along the direction of the air-flow, nondistributed sounds are produced with a constriction that extends only a short distance in this direction. (Chomsky and Halle, 1968, p. 312)

Thus, apical and retroflex stops were opposed to laminal and nonretroflex stops as − *distributed* to + *distributed.* Chomsky and Halle also characterized the distinction between Polish "hard" and "soft" dentals in terms of the feature *distributed:*

> It is this longer stricture that accounts for the striking hushing quality that is observed in Polish 'soft' dentals. (1968, p. 314)

Chomsky and Halle contrasted Polish soft dentals with the Russian "soft" /s/, which does not have this hushing quality:

> It is formed with a much shorter stricture and thus must be regarded as −distributed. (1968, p. 314)

The feature *delayed release* as opposed to *instantaneous release* Chomsky and Halle described as affecting:

> . . . only sounds produced with closure of the vocal tract . . . During delayed release turbulence is generated in the vocal tract so that the release phase of the affricates is acoustically quite similar to the cognate fricative. (1968, p. 318)

PART II
A Comparison
of the
Feature System
Developed in Grundzüge
with
Earlier Classifications
and
Those of Preliminaries,
Fundamentals,
and
The Sound Pattern
of English

With Jakobson's *Observations sur le classement phonologique des consonnes* (1938), any mutual influence that Trubetzkoy and Jakobson may have had on each other ends. *Observations* was Jakobson's last publication before Trubetzkoy's death and the last one before Trubetzkoy's culminating work, *Grundzüge der Phonologie* (1939).

In tracing the development and sources of the theory of distinctive features, a comparison between Jakobson's earlier work and Trubetzkoy's subsequent *Grundzüge* is relevant. It is important to establish what Trubetzkoy's *Grundzüge* had in common with Jakobson's later work and how it must have influenced Jakobson and the feature framework reformulated by Chomsky and Halle.

In Trubetzkoy's *Die phonologischen Systeme* (1931a), the basic split in oppositions had been between vowels and consonants. The prosodic oppositions formed a major class in the vowel system. In *Grundzüge* (1939), Trubetzkoy split his classifications three ways: consonantal, vocalic, and prosodic. The basis for his separation of the prosodic properties from the vocalic properties was the establishment of the prosodic unit. In discussing the prosodic unit, Trubetzkoy claimed that it was not entirely identical with the syllable, but largely so. Prosodic properties here were thus transferred from the vowels and became properties of the prosodic unit as a whole.[65]

The classification of distinctive oppositions as it appeared in *Grundzüge* differed in several ways from the classification as it appeared in *Die phonologischen Systeme*. One way was the aforementioned three-way split in types of oppositions: vocalic, consonantal, and prosodic. This contrasts with the earlier two-way split between consonantal and vocalic oppositions.

Also gone from *Grundzüge* is any allusion to "natural classes" *(Wesensverwandtschaftsgruppen)*. Instead there is a classification of oppositions that seems to draw vowels and consonants closer together. As in *Die phonologischen Systeme,* Trubetzkoy continued to view the classification of consonants as more difficult and complex than that of vowels. He maintained that this was because of the natural asymmetry generally existing between vowels and consonants in terms of number of occurrences in any given system. It may be added that the basic configuration of the oral cavity in the production of vowels and consonants differs sufficiently to add to this disparity. The Polish scholar

Kuryłowicz (1967) also underscored the importance of the difference in number between vowels and consonants and its possible
effect on the classification. Martinet (1949) called attention to the
second point.

In *Grundzüge* the consonants were contrasted to the vowels
as follows. Important for the consonants was a closure-aperture
movement with an articulatory maximum between the two
points. In contrast, an aperture-closure movement was important
for the vowels, with an articulatory minimum between the two
points. Put somewhat differently, "what characterizes a consonant is the production of an obstruction and the overcoming of such
an obstruction" while "a vowel is characterized by the absence of
any obstruction, i.e., practically speaking, by various degrees
of aperture" (Trubetzkoy, 1939/1969, p. 94).[66]

Chomsky and Halle paralleled this articulatory correlate in
The Sound Patterns of English when they divided features into
sonorant, vocalic, and consonantal as major class features:

> Reduced to the most rudimentary terms, the behavior of the vocal
> tract in speech can be described as an alternation of closing and
> opening . . . . Each of the major class features—sonorant, vocalic,
> consonantal—focuses on a different aspect of the open v. close phase.
> (1968, p. 301 ff.)

The Trubetzkoyan distinction between vowels and consonants can also be represented by a binary contrast: +/− an *obstruction* or +/− *absence of an obstruction*. In accordance with
such a binary contrast, Trubetzkoy considered properties or
features pertaining to consonants (+*obstruction*) and to vowels
(−*obstruction*) as specifically consonantal or specifically vocalic,
respectively.

In addition to two separate sets of features that were specifically consonantal or specifically vocalic, Trubetzkoy established
two other major classes shared by vowels and consonants: *properties of localization* and *properties of resonance*.

One of the main differences between the Trubetzkoyan and
Jakobsonian classifications is that Trubetzkoy had two separate
sets of properties which, to the exclusion of each other, were specifically consonantal or specifically vocalic. The Jakobsonian classification did not make such a distinction, and the same set of
features applied to both consonants and vowels.

According to Trubetzkoy, any phonological system was analyzable in terms of the above "three coordinates to vowel or consonant quality." Of these three coordinates, expressed in aperture or obstruction, localization, and resonance features, not all had to be present in every vowel or consonant phoneme. However, any feature which was distinctive for a vowel or a consonant phoneme had to belong to one of the above three classes. Table 5 represents this basic classificatory framework.

A comparison of the classification of *Grundzüge* with that of the earlier *Die phonologischen Systeme* reveals several differences. One, as noted earlier, was the separation of the prosodic oppositions from the vocalic oppositions. In addition, a considerable unification process between vowels and consonants took place. Furthermore, some of the individual oppositions were shifted in classification (cf. above, p. 72 ff.).

THE VOWELS: APERTURE AND TIMBRE

Even though Trubetzkoy had established common coordinates for vowels and consonants, he continued to discuss vowel and consonant properties separately with respect to all three coordinates.

Trubetzkoy endeavored to establish acoustic correlates for his classification and at least in part replaced earlier articulatory terminology. His rationale had been that "the linguist is interested in the acoustic effect," and that "modern phonetics ascribes more consistency and uniformity to the acoustic effect than to the articulatory movements producing it" (1939/1969, p. 92). In an attempt to follow acoustic terminology for vowels, he coined the term "properties based on degree of sonority or saturation" for "aperture" oppositions, and "properties of timbre" for the articulatory term "properties of localization." Trubetzkoy maintained that "acoustically these properties correspond to various gaps in a series of partial tones *(Teiltone)*": front vowels show an increase in the higher, and a suppression in the lower partial tones; conversely, the higher partial tones are the ones which are suppressed in the back vowels (see below, p. 113).

Trubetzkoy maintained that for the vowels the coordinates of aperture and timbre are more closely related to each other than to the third coordinate, resonance, In *Die phonologischen Systeme,*

Table 5. The three basic coordinates to vowel and consonant qualities of *Grundzüge*

Obstruction (first coordinate, separating consonants and vowels)

+obstruction Consonants *Articulatory correlate:* production of an obstruction and overcoming such an obstruction in the oral cavity
Properties or features related thereto: properties based on the manner of overcoming an obstruction

−obstruction Vowels *Articulatory correlate:* absence of an obstruction
Properties or features related thereto: properties based on degree of aperture

Localization (second coordinate to vowel and consonant quality)

+localization Consonants *Articulatory correlate:* localization (place) of different types of obstruction or the different modes of overcoming an obstruction
Properties related thereto: properties of localization

+localization Vowels *Articulatory correlate:* localization of different degrees of aperture
Properties related thereto: properties of localization (= timbre)

Resonance (third coordinate to vowel and consonant quality)

+resonance Consonants and vowels *Acoustic correlates:* specific acoustic features in the production of vowels and consonants related to the establishment and the disruption of the connection with a second resonator
Properties related thereto: properties of resonance

aperture and timbre had belonged to one major class (see above, p. 72 ff.). In *Grundzüge,* he set up three basic types of vowel system: (1) a linear system, (2) a quadrangular system, and (3) a triangular system.

In this classification the categories of vowel systems did not essentially change from the earlier classificatory system of *Zur allgemeinen Theorie der phonologischen Vokalsysteme* (1929a). An exception is that systems, such as that of Adyghe, a language of the Northern Caucasus, which only have aperture as a distinctive opposition were now labeled "linear systems."

It is further noteworthy, in a comparison with the earlier *Zur allgemeinen Theorie* and *Die phonologischen Systeme,* that in *Grundzüge* Trubetzkoy attempted to establish the acoustic *and* the articulatory correlates for his oppositions. Even though he had used acoustic terms for vowel oppositions in *Zur allgemeinen Theorie,* he did not define the terms acoustically. The term "acoustic" in this context is to be understood as impressionistically acoustic.

The pivotal opposition members or "terms" in the Trubetzkoyan classification of vocalic oppositions were the maximally open vowels, since these were the determining factor in feature redundancy. The primacy of the aperture opposition for vowels had already been stressed in *Zur allgemeinen Theorie* (see above, p. 69 ff.). In *Grundzüge* the maximally open vowel took on additional importance with respect to phonological redundancy: if its opposing member was unrounded with respect to timbre, the second coordinate to vowel quality, the opposition of rounding became irrelevant for the entire system. The opposition of tongue position (that is, back/front = grave/acute = palatovelar) remained the only one which was distinctive. If, on the other hand, the maximally open vowel has a rounded vowel as its opposing member in terms of timbre, the front/back opposition becomes redundant for the entire system.

This rule was also tacitly observed in the subsequent Jakobsonian classification, where it found expression in the economy metric based on the number of pluses and minuses. It can be derived from a general rule already expressed by Trubetzkoy, namely, that the maximally open vowel never contains more distinctions with respect to timbre (gravity and flatness in terms of Jakobsonian features) than the less open vowels. An analysis in terms of timbre would therefore yield the same classification for

Jakobson and for Trubetzkoy. Differences in approach, however, can be found in an analysis of the vertical parameter, represented by the aperture opposition for Trubetzkoy and by the compact/ diffuse opposition for Jakobson.

Trubetzkoy's above two rules, relating to the primacy of the aperture opposition and to the dependency in the choice of the opposition of timbre (that is, either gravity or flatness) on the maximally open vowel, can be illustrated by the vowel system for some archaic Monte Negran dialects of the Serbo-Croatian language group (where the Protoslavic semivowels did not develop into an "a" but into an "æ"). The assumption here is that the factual data presented are correct. Trubetzkoy gave six vowels for that system: a, æ, o, e, u, i. According to the above two statements, only one possibility for the classification of that system exists: it is broken down into one ternary opposition (aperture) and one binary opposition (gravity), as in Figure 5.

While Trubetzkoy made the aperture opposition primary, Jakobson did not explicitly state any requirement regarding the primacy of the aperture (compactness/diffuseness) opposition in actual classification. (It is interesting to note that Jakobson did acknowledge this requirement with respect to language acquisition in his *Kindersprache, Aphasie und allgemeine Lautgesetze* (1942/1962d).) Instead, Jakobson strove for as close a binary classification as possible. The above statement needs to be qualified, however: exposed to the conflict of a choice between minimal number of features versus strict adherence to the principle of binarity, Jakobson vacillated over time. For example, at the time of *Preliminaries to Speech Analysis* (Jakobson, Fant, and Halle, 1952), the choice of a minimal number of features still appeared to be his primary classificatory criterion.

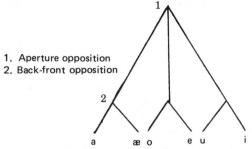

1. Aperture opposition
2. Back-front opposition

a   æ o   e u   i

Figure 5. Trubetzkoy's classification of Monte Negran dialects broken down into one ternary opposition (aperture) and one binary opposition (gravity).

The opposition compact/diffuse, and for that matter, the opposition grave/acute, was therefore treated as ternary. In *Toward a Logical Description of Languages in Their Phonemic Aspect* (Jakobson, Cherry, and Halle, 1953), the opposition compact/diffuse was split, and the binarity principle appears to become primary.[67] At the time of *Fundamentals of Language* (Jakobson and Halle, 1956), the feature compact/diffuse again was viewed as ternary.

The binary approach to analysis à la Jakobson (without a split in the compact/diffuse dichotomy) presents a problem with the front-low /æ/ in the vowel system of the Monte Negran dialects. Without such a vowel—that is, if the system were represented by five vowels (/i, e, a, o, u/)—a binary analysis would be no problem. Even though three degrees of aperture are present, the oppositions of timbre, front-back, and rounded-unrounded (that is, gravity and flatness) could, contrary to Trubetzkoy, be utilized. The opposition of aperture could thus be represented as binary, as shown in Table 6. Such an analysis is in fact found in *Preliminaries* (p. 43) in conjunction with /ə/. There both the opposition /o-a/ and the opposition /u-ə/ were analyzed as one of the flat/plain (= rounded/unrounded).

Table 6.   Five-vowel system represented as binary, modeled on *Preliminaries* (1952)

	/i/	/e/	/a/	/o/	/u/
Front/back	+	+	−	−	−
Compact/diffuse	−	+	+	+	−
Rounded/unrounded				−	+

However, this was not the only way in which Jakobson analyzed a five-vowel system of the above type. For example, in *On the Identification of Phonemic Entities* (1949c, p. 421), the vowel system of Serbo-Croatian was analyzed by means of two oppositions, saturation (= compact/diffuse) and gravity, as shown in Table 7. Here saturation was obviously ternary and gravity was obviously binary. The resulting system was thus in accord with that permissible by the Trubetzkoyan classification (but see below, p. 103).

In Toward a *Logical Description of Languages in Their Phonemic Aspect* Jakobson described the five-vowel system of Russian, with the opposition compact/diffuse split and the

Table 7. Jakobson's analysis of the Serbo-Croatian five-vowel system by means of two oppositions

	/i/	/u/	/e/	/o/	/a/
Saturation	−	−	±	±	+
Gravity	−	+	−	+	

From Jakobson, 1949c, p. 421.

stressed vowel system shown in Table 8 (Jakobson, Cherry, and Halle, 1953, p. 454).

It is interesting to note that the analysis of the stressed vowel system in Russian represented a change from an earlier conception for both Jakobson and Trubetzkoy. In *Die phonologischen Systeme* (p. 100 ff.; also p. 101, n.4), on the advice of Jakobson, Trubetzkoy had analyzed the Russian vocalic system using two oppositions, aperture and rounding, on the basis of the common denominator for all positional variants:

The Russian vowel phonemes are divided into rounded /u,o/ and unrounded /i,e,a/ vowels; if they occur between two palatalized consonants, they belong in part to the series of back vowels /u,o,a/, in part to the series of mid vowels /i = phonetic ɨ, e = phonetic æ /. In the remaining positions /u,o/ and /a/ belong to the back series, /i/ and /e/ to the front series. Accordingly, only lip rounding (and degree of aperture) are phonologically relevant for Russian vowels, while tongue position is entirely dependent on the phonetic context. (A similar picture is also seen in the Polish vowel system.)

In *Grundzüge*, the oppositions of timbre would be considered fused (1939/1969, p. 110 ff., and below, p. 103), since both rounding and gravity applied. In *Logical Description*, Jakobson used the gravity feature alone. It thus seems that, compared to Trubetzkoy's *Die phonologischen Systeme*, both scholars had arrived at a greater degree of abstraction.

Table 8. Jakobson's analysis of the five-vowel system of Russian

	/u/	/o/	/e/	/i/	/a/
Compact	−	−	−	−	+
Diffuse	+	−	−	+	
Grave	+	+	−	−	

From Jakobson, Cherry, and Halle, 1953, p. 454.

A fourth classification is found in *Preliminaries* (p. 44). In acknowledging the joint presence of two opposite features in one phoneme, Jakobson, Fant, and Halle reduced the above five vowels to two oppositions (actually the system also included /a/), as shown in Table 9.

The fourth classification in particular points up the general lability of the compact/diffuse opposition. The vowels of mid aperture are included here under compactness.

While in the above example of *Preliminaries,* gravity was essentially considered as a ternary opposition, Jakobson in *Fundamentals* wrote: "Among the inherent features, *only* the vocalic distinction compact/diffuse often represents a higher number of terms, mostly three" (1952, p. 48; emphasis added).

As mentioned, within the Trubetzkoyan framework, it would have been possible to classify a five-vowel system like the one discussed earlier (/i,u,a,e,o/) in one way only. A Trubetzkoyan classification would not have been quite identical with any of the feature specifications resulting from the Jakobsonian analyses. Such a classification would have come closest to the one found in Jakobson's *Identification* and reproduced in Table 8. One major difference would reside in the overtly gradual character of the opposition of aperture as opposed to the Jakobsonian ± notation, indicating the joint presence of features in his analysis.

A second difference is that Jakobson regarded the opposition of rounding as redundant in the example given in *Identification.* Trubetzkoy, on the other hand, would have considered it a component of a fused unit: in those cases where both the features *front* and *unrounded* and *back* and *rounded,* respectively, occur together distinctively in all phonemes concerned, these two oppositions of timbre could not be separated. Trubetzkoy considered them a "fused unit" and opposed to each other as logically equipollent. He called the back-rounded member of that opposition "maximally dark," and the front-unrounded member, the

Table 9.   The Jakobson, Fant, and Halle analysis of the five-vowel (plus schwa) Russian system reduced to two oppositions

	/o/	/a/	/e/	/u/	/ə/	/i/
Compact/diffuse	+	+	+	−	−	−
Grave/acute	+	±	−	+	±	−

From Jakobson, Fant, and Halle, 1952, p. 44.

"maximally clear" vowel. He noted that even though these two oppositions do not frequently coalesce in quadrangular systems, they do frequently coalesce in triangular systems. The maximally open vowel in triangular systems stands outside of any class of timbre. In other words, timbre is redundant for /a/ in such a system.

Because of Trubetzkoy's above conception, gravity and flatness were considered a fused unit in the case of the above five-vowel system and neither feature was considered redundant (see Table 10).

To come back to the analysis of the six-vowel system of the Monte Negran dialects, the Trubetzkoyan classification allowed only one possible interpretation (see Figure 5). Jakobson, in according ternary status to the opposition compact/diffuse, would have arrived at the same analysis as Trubetzkoy, although with a change in labeling.

With the subsequent split of the compact/diffuse opposition in the Jakobsonian classification, a second possibility of analysis became available. The Monte Negran vowel system could now be analyzed into three binary oppositions. The first solution thus adhered to the principle of economy relative to the number of features, the second solution to the principle of binarity.

It can be expected that if the two systems were analyzed in the Chomsky and Halle feature framework, they would be analyzed in terms of the features high, low, and back, as shown in Table 11.

In summary, the differences between Trubetzkoy and Jakobson as they relate to the above classification are twofold: 1) they are based on rules established by Trubetzkoy and not followed by Jakobson (such rules would include, for example, the primacy of aperture in a classificatory matrix), and 2) they are the consequence of development in feature theory post-dating Trubetzkoy (for example, the split of the compact/diffuse opposition). It would

Table 10.   Trubetzkoyan analysis of a five-vowel system[a]

	/i/	/u/	/e/	/o/	/a/
Aperture	−	−	=	=	+
Front/back	+	−	+	−	
Unrounded/rounded	+	−	+	−	

[a] The "=" sign here denotes gradualness rather than joint presence.

Table 11. Chomsky and Halle expected analysis

Feature	Monte Negran (six-vowel system)						Serbo-Croatian (five-vowel system)				
	/i/	/u/	/e/	/o/	/æ/	/a/	/i/	/u/	/e/	/o/	/a/
High	+	+	−	−	−	−	+	+	−	−	−
Low	−	−	−	−	+	+	−	−	−	−	+
Back	−	+	−	+	−	+	−	+	−	+	

follow from what has been said that a feature analysis within the Jakobsonian tradition was more flexible than within the Trubetzkoyan system.

As mentioned earlier, a major difference between the two classifications related to the first coordinate to vowel and consonant quality. This coordinate was one of obstruction, and the oppositions relating to obstruction were either considered specifically vocalic or specifically consonantal and did not overlap. Thus the opposition compact/diffuse (= aperture) never extended to the consonants in the Trubetzkoyan classification. With respect to the second coordinate to vowel and consonantal quality relating to properties of localization, also called properties of timbre, a close tie was expressed in the Trubetzkoyan classification between the back/front opposition (grave/acute) and the opposition of rounding (flat/plain).[68] (This is evident, for example, from their parallelism in occurrence, and the special nomenclature associated with cases in which the two features coalesced in terms of "maximally dark" and "maximally clear.") The close relationship between the two features was also recognized by Jakobson, who termed timbre "tonality." However, in the Jakobsonian classification, a third tonality feature was added that had not yet occurred among the Trubetzkoyan oppositions of localizations. The new opposition was sharp/plain.

Jakobson used the terms "optimally acute" and "optimally grave," respectively, (Jakobson, Fant, and Halle, 1952, p. 33ff., 46) for what Trubetzkoy had labeled "maximally clear" and "maximally dark." Jakobson further proposed that if one opposition were present only in the vowels and the other only in the consonants, the oppositions grave/acute and flat/plain could be coalesced (Jakobson, Fant, and Halle, 1952, p. 34).

The close relationship between aperture and timbre or tonality features was also recognized by Jakobson when he observed that the timbre or tonality features have a propensity for diffuse vowels (Jakobson, Fant, and Halle, 1952:34; see also Jakobson, 1938).

Chomsky and Halle also recognized the special relationship between timbre and tonality features and the propensity for these features to occur in diffuse vowels. They captured these generalities in *The Sound Pattern of English* (1968) in their theory of markedness, as represented by marking conventions VI through XI (p. 403 ff.) shown in Figure 6.

In Trubetzkoy's *Die phonologischen Systeme* (1931a, p. 100 ff.), the opposition of tension was mentioned as a possible third class of oppositions in the natural class of oppositions of quality. This is not mentioned for the vowels in *Grundzüge*. Instead, there is what Trubetzkoy called an "opposition of closeness" (1939/1969, p. 109) in addition to the aperture opposition discussed earlier.

With respect to properties of resonance, Trubetzkoy's third coordinate to vowel and consonant quality, no substantial change

$$\text{(VI)}\quad [u\ \text{low}] \rightarrow \begin{cases} [+\text{low}] \;/\; \begin{bmatrix} \overline{u\ \text{back}} \\ u\ \text{round} \end{bmatrix} & \text{(a)} \\ [-\text{low}] & \text{(b)} \end{cases}$$

Where:

$$\text{(VII)}\quad [+\text{low}] \rightarrow [-\text{high}]$$

$$\text{(VIII)}\quad [u\ \text{high}] \rightarrow [+\text{high}]$$

$$\text{(IX)}\quad [+\text{high}] \rightarrow [-\text{low}]$$

And:

$$\text{(X)}\quad [u\ \text{back}] \rightarrow [+\text{back}] \;/\; \begin{bmatrix} \underline{} \\ +\text{low} \end{bmatrix}$$

$$\text{(XI)}\quad [u\ \text{round}] \rightarrow \begin{cases} [\alpha\ \text{round}] \;/\; \begin{bmatrix} \overline{\alpha\ \text{back}} \\ -\text{low} \end{bmatrix} & \text{(a)} \\ [-\text{round}] \;/\; \begin{bmatrix} \underline{} \\ +\text{low} \end{bmatrix} & \text{(b)} \end{cases}$$

Figure 6. Chomsky-Halle application of markedness to timbre and tonality features. (From Chomsky and Halle, 1968, p. 403 ff.).

had taken place in *Grundzüge* when compared to their earlier classification in *Die phonologischen Systeme*.

It should be pointed out here that Trubetzkoy's resonance oppositions did not coincide with what Jakobson, Fant, and Halle in *Preliminaries* called "resonance features." Trubetzkoy had stated three coordinates to vowel and consonant quality in *Grundzüge*, after first setting up a distinction between vocalic, consonantal, and prosodic features. In contrast, Jakobson, Fant, and Halle differentiated between inherent features and prosodic features but did not discuss their prosodic features. (These are discussed later, in *Fundamentals*.) Inherent features are applied to both consonants and vowels. Within these features Jakobson, Fant, and Halle distinguished between: 1) *the fundamental source features* (vocalic/nonvocalic, consonantal/nonconsonantal, which separated vowels, consonants, liquids, and glides), and 2) *secondary consonantal source features,* classified as the envelope features (continuant/interrupted, checked/unchecked) and the stridency feature (strident/mellow) as *primary source features*. The secondary consonantal source features also included the voicing feature, attributable to a supplementary source.

The *resonance features* were listed as a separate class and included compactness, the three tonality features (gravity, flatness, and sharpness), and tenseness, as well as nasalization, attributable to a supplementary resonator.

Resonance features in *Preliminaries* included those which in *Grundzüge* had been listed in connection with the first coordinate to vowel quality (the compactness feature) and the second coordinate (the timbre features of gravity and flatness but not sharpness). As indicated above, the tenseness feature apparently had been dropped for vowels in *Grundzüge* and replaced by the *closeness feature*. Nasalization was the only one Trubetzkoy considered a resonance feature, and thus the only one on which the Trubetzkoyan and Jakobsonian classifications agreed as to what constituted a resonance feature.

For comparative purposes, Table 12 presents the Trubetzkoyan classificatory schema as it appeared in *Grundzüge* along with that of Jakobson, Fant, and Halle as it appeared in *Preliminaries* with emphasis on the correspondences between the Jakobsonian resonance features in the Trubetzkoyan vowel schema.

Comparing the basic classificatory schemata of Trubetzkoy and Jakobson it becomes obvious that different criteria had been

Table 12.   Correspondences of Jakobson, Fant, and Halle (1952) resonance features with Trubetzkoy (1939) vowel features

Preliminaries to Speech Analysis	*Grundzüge der Phonologie*
Fundamental source features	Obstruction
Vocalic-nonvocalic	*Vowels*/consonants

Consonantal-nonconsonantal
  (separating the vowels, consonants,
  liquids, and glides)
	Aperture (= compactness)

Secondary consonantal source features	Localization
Envelope features	*Vowels*/consonants
Continued-interrupted	Timbre
Checked-unchecked	rounded-unrounded (flatness)
Stridency feature	Front-back (gravity)
Strident-mellow	
Voicing feature	
Voiced-unvoiced	
Resonance features	Resonance
Compact/diffuse	*Vowels*/consonants
Tonality features	Nasalization (= nasalization)
Gravity (front-back)	
Flatness (rounding)	
Sharpness (palatalization)	
Tenseness	
Nasal(ization)	

used in the two classifications. Trubetzkoy required a hierarchy (at least for vowels) between his first coordinate to consonant and vowel quality obstruction, and his second coordinate, relating to localization. Within his localization features, the features of flatness and gravity were also rank ordered. His third coordinate to vowel and consonant quality, relating to resonance, was not considered as closely linked to the former two as the first two coordinates were to each other. In *Preliminaries*, which was written from the point of view of instrumental acoustics, no reason is stated for why the classificatory schema was sub-divided in the way it was.[69] Nevertheless, the feature classifica-tion of *Preliminaries* appears to follow some covert principles:

1. The first subdivision supplies the basic elements to which further features relate
2. The second division applies to the consonants resulting from the first division

3. The third division covers those features which are shared by all the elements resultant from the first division

The voicing feature, which is also listed in the second division (secondary consonantal source features), could be considered an exception. However, justification for its inclusion into this subdivision rather than the third subdivision of resonance seems to be given in *Preliminaries* by the following statement:

> Vowels are normally voiced. It is still questionable whether there are languages in which parallel to the consonantal opposition voiced-voiceless there actually is a similar distinctive opposition of voice and murmured vowels . . . Either the vocal murmur is not a distinctive feature and functions merely as a border mark, or it may be a concomitant of the tense-lax opposition. (Jakobson, Fant, and Halle, 1952, p. 26)

The opposition checked/unchecked is also listed under secondary consonantal source features, though it probably would have to be considered an exception to the second principle stated above. Also, the Jakobsonian compactness feature intersects with both the first and second subdivision of the Trubetzkoyan classification, since it refers to aperture in vowels and to localization or place of articulation in consonants.

When the Jakobsonian classifications of *Preliminaries* and *Fundamentals* are compared, the following changes can be observed: in *Fundamentals,* after an initial division of features into prosodic and inherent features:

> . . . all the inherent features are divided into two classes that might be termed sonority and tonality features. The sonority features utilize the amount and concentration of energy in the spectrum and in time. The tonality features involve the ends of the frequency spectrum. (Jakobson and Halle, 1952, p. 29)

The following division for sonority features is given in *Fundamentals* (p. 29 ff.):

Vocalic/nonvocalic
Consonantal/nonconsonantal
Compact/diffuse
Tense/lax
Voiced/voiceless
Nasal/oral
Discontinuous/continuant
Strident/mellow
Checked/unchecked

And for tonality features:

Grave/acute
Flat/plain
Sharp/plain

The tonality features in *Fundamentals* now corresponded to the Trubetzkoyan second coordinate to vowel and consonant quality relating to localization features (to the exclusion of the sharpness feature) with regard to the vowels. Compared to the classification in *Preliminaries* it is obvious that the classificatory criteria for *Fundamentals* have changed in terms of the earlier and subsequent subdivisions.

THE CONSONANTS

A comparison of Trubetzkoy's position on the classification of consonants with that of Jakobson reveals several differences. As mentioned earlier, Trubetzkoy seemed to have been familiar with the Jakobsonian binary classification of *Observations sur le classement phonologique des consonnes* (1938) at the time he wrote the section on consonants in *Grundzüge* (1939). He adopted the Jakobsonian opposition strident/mellow into his own classification (Jakobson, 1938, p. 277; Trubetzkoy 1939/1969, p. 127 ff.) although with some differences in application which are discussed below. He further added the opposition flat/plain, which Jakobson (1938) had not yet included in his classification. As discussed below, *Grundzüge* has some overlap between the opposition flat/plain, strident/mellow, and the Jakobsonian opposition grave/acute. Retroflexes and labiovelar consonants had not been part of the classification in *Observations*. They were grouped into the opposition flat/plain in *Grundzüge*.

As discussed earlier, Trubetzkoy in *Grundzüge* had organized his features along three coordinates to vowel and consonant quality. The resultant classification included features that applied exclusively to vowels or to consonants. These exclusive features belonged to Trubetzkoy's first coordinate. In addition, other features applied equally to vowels and consonants (see Table 12). These features related to localization and resonance. Below, these features and their relevance to the subsequent development of feature theory are discussed.

Localization Features for Consonants

Basic Series   Based on the criteria of naturalness and generality or universality, Trubetzkoy set up four basic consonant classes: labials, apicals, gutturals, and sibilants. Naturalness, as the term was used by Trubetzkoy, related to naturalness of position of the articulating organs. Thus, the universality of these sounds, according to Trubetzkoy, was explicable in terms of their "naturalness."

Of the four basic classes the most universal were the labials, apicals, and gutturals. These were followed by the sibilants. In addition to these four "most universal" series, another series of four were also considered basic: laterals, labiovelars, palatals, and laryngeals.

A series was considered basic if its consonant members stood in a relation of heterogeneous multilateral opposition to each other (cf. above, p. 52 ff.). This meant that their relationship to each other had to be opaque and could not be analyzed further into binary oppositions. If a binary relationship could be established, the series was not considered basic but belonged to what was considered a related series.

A basic series was termed a "related series" when it stood in binary relationship to another basic series. A binary relationship between two basic series was supported by neutralizability and similarity in physical correlates. According to Trubetzkoy, neutralization of an opposition presented convincing evidence that an opposition was actually binary and not only logically binary.

Trubetzkoy found that binary relations exist quite frequently between the apical and the sibilant series in a given language. Their relatedness was also supported by the articulatory correlates of the two series which consist in the similarity of the upper and back portion of the oral resonator in their production. Where binary relations could be established, the apical and sibilant series were not considered two separate basic localization series; instead, they were considered related series.

Based on neutralizability, binary relations could frequently be established between the palatals and velars and between palatals and dentals. Where neutralization played a role, the palatal series was not considered a basic, but a related series.

Binary relations were also found between the velars and the

labiovelars. Both these consonant classes were mentioned as basic series.

Based on observations relating to languages in general, Trubetzkoy thus posited eight possible basic series. He maintained that the number of basic series which could be established for any given language would be in all probability smaller than the number established in terms of phonological universals. He based this conclusion on language-specific observations that comprised actual occurrences of these consonant classes in a given language as well as their contextual or distributional behavior including their neutralizability.

This distinction between basic and related series illuminates an elusive difference pertaining to opposition relationships between the Trubetzkoyan classification of *Grundzüge* and the Jakobsonian one of *Preliminaries* and *Fundamentals*. Depending on the contextual constraints which governed a (universal) basic series in a given language, its universal status as a basic series could change. Such a distinction was not made in the Jakobsonian classification: once an opposition relationship was established in terms of "universal features" it did not change its status.

The following example illustrates this point. For Trubetzkoy, if a given language has the four consonant classes these could be handled as follows in terms of basic series:

(1) Labials	Apicals	Palatals	Gutturals
(2) Labials	{ Apicals Palatals		Gutturals
(3) Labials	Apicals		{ Gutturals Palatals

Depending on the distributional criteria within a language either three or four basic series would exist. In the above instance, based on contextual constraints and naturalization, the palatal and the apical, or the guttural and the palatal, could be considered related series.

In the Jakobsonian classification, on the other hand, all three above possibilities would be handled by the features compactness and gravity without regard to the behavior of these sounds in a given language.

It should also be pointed out that the "series of localization" of *Grundzüge* were not entirely equivalent to the points of articulation parameter. Assignment to a series of localization was governed by the symmetry and coherence of the entire phonological system. Thus, if a language had the oppositions /z-s/, /ž-š/, and /h-x/, the opposition /h-x/ was considered as belonging to the same localization series because of systemic pressure *(Systemzwang)* even though /h/ and /x/ differ in point of articulation in addition to voicing. Trubetzkoy illustrated instances of systemic pressure from Czech and Slovak (1939/1969, p. 125). The inclusion of oppositions into a basic series based on systemic pressure represents a refinement over his earlier position in *Die phonologischen Systeme* (1931a), where oppositions of localizations had been equated with oppositions based on points of articulation (see above, p. 74).

Related Series   In addition to the eight potentially basic series of localization, Trubetzkoy also set up "equipollent related series." His rationale for doing this was that in some languages "two series occur for some of these basic series" (1939/1969, p. 125). According to Trubetzkoy such series can be seen as a split in the given basic series and are definable in binary terms vis-à-vis the respective basic series. Neutralization in this case was not seen as a prerequisite for establishing binarity. Such related series can be illustrated by the co-existence of labials and labiodentals in a labiodental series, the existence, in addition to an alveolar series, of an interdental in the apical series and a predorsal and postdorsal in the guttural series. The status of this type of related series never changed: language-universal versus language-specific considerations did not play a role here.

The following general observations can be made in comparing the basic and related series of the Trubetzkoyan classification to the Jakobsonian classification involving the same sounds.

First, Trubetzkoy did not follow Jakobson in establishing the two oppositions grave/acute and compact/diffuse for the consonants despite the fact that, by his own acknowledgment, he knew about the Jakobsonian classification in *Observations*. Trubetzkoy's classification consisted instead of essentially independent basic series. This distinction constitutes one of the major and fundamental differences between the Trubetzkoyan and Jakobsonian classification and affected both the Jakobsonian and the Trubetzkoyan classificatory system in its entirety.

The establishment of these series by Trubetzkoy were related to questions of naturalness in terms of articulation as well as of generality or universality of occurrence. The existence of these series in any given language related first to their actual presence and second to their contextual or distributional behavior in that language.

Although the Jakobsonian features had been posited as universal features, no distinction had been made between sounds that are more general than others. For example, the fact that palatals universally occur less frequently than labials, apicals, or gutturals was not expressed in that classification. (Jakobson considered such variables in his *Kindersprache, Aphasie und allgemeine Lautgesetze* (1962, pp. 328–401) but not as a direct aspect of his distinctive feature theory). Certain distributional relationships which had played a role for Trubetzkoy were also obscured in the subsequent Jakobsonian classification.

Second, even though Trubetzkoy adopted the Jakobsonian opposition strident/mellow, his use of it did not have the same range of application as for Jakobson. The lack of a full equivalency was partially attributable to the establishment of the basic series in the Trubetzkoyan classification that included more classes than the labials, apicals, palatals, and velars.

Third, Trubetzkoy accommodated the retroflexes and labiovelars. It will be recalled that, by establishing the opposition flat/plain, their classification had been left undecided in Jakobson's *Observations*. Both the opposition flat/plain and the opposition strident/mellow could occur as ternary oppositions in the Trubetzkoyan classification. For example, the distinction between /s-š-ŝ/ was viewed in terms of different degrees of stridency. The distinction between palatals, prevelars, and postvelars, or alveolars, interdentals, and palatals, was viewed as related to different degrees of flatness (see Trubetzkoy, 1939/1969, p. 128 ff.).

In reference to the first point above, it is clear that the Jakobsonian features of gravity and compactness were not adequate to differentiate all of Trubetzkoy's basic series. This is particularly true for the basic series relating to back consonants. This inadequacy was also pointed out by Chomsky and Halle. It constituted a consideration for the replacement of the gravity and compactness features by the features high, low, and back (Chomsky and Halle, 1968, p. 308). Within the Jakobsonian framework, it had not been possible to distinguish equally between the velars, uvulars, and pharyngeals based on their points of articulation. Instead, in the words of Chomsky and Halle (1968, p. 308) the "subsidiary feature of stridency" had to be used.

In the Trubetzkoyan framework of basic series, these back consonants had all been distinguished based on the same parameter (localization) and had been of equal status with respect to localization.

In reference to the second point above and the feature stridency, already discussed (see above, p. 77 ff.), is the fact that Jakobson in *Observations* analyzed the four consonant classes, labials, dentals, palatals, and velars, by the two features grave/acute and compact/diffuse, based on the volume and shape of the oral resonators. He divided each of the classes into two series each and then distinguished among each of the two series by the strident/mellow opposition. The stridency feature was also used

Table 13.   Correspondences of the feature mellow/strident[a] for Jakobson (*Observations*, 1938, *Preliminaries*, 1952) and Trubetzkoy (*Grundzüge*, 1939)

Jakobson	Trubetzkoy
Labials	Labials
Bilabials (M)	Bilabials /b, p, m/ (M)
Labiodentals (S)	Labiodentals /v, f, p/ (S)
Dentals	
Linguadentals /θ/(M)	
s-sounds (*sifflantes*)/s/(S)	
Palatals	
Palatals (M)	Sibilants /s/ (M), /š/ (S)
š-sounds (*chuintants*) (S)	
Gutturals	Gutturals
Velars (M)	Prevelar /x/ (M)
Uvulars (S)	Postvelar /x̌/ (S)
Stops	
Stops (M)	
Affricates (S)	
	Laryngeals
	True laryngeals /h/ (M)
	Pharyngeals /ḥ/ (S)
Liquids[b]	

[a] M, mellow; S, strident.
[b] Added in *Preliminaries*.

to distinguish between stops and affricates. (For the Jakobsonian physical correlates of stridency as stated in *Observations* and *Preliminaries*, see above, p. 84 ff.). Trubetzkoy had accepted the Jakobsonian stridency opposition, simply opposing the strident sounds to the mellow sounds as "more audible to less audible."

As pointed out earlier, the four consonant classes which Jakobson differentiated by the gravity and compactness features were not identical with the sum of the Trubetzkoyan basic series but rather represented a selection therefrom.

The application of the stridency feature is somewhat wider in range in the Trubetzkoyan than in the Jakobsonian framework. This is because it applies not only to the above four consonant classes differentiated by Jakobsonian by gravity and compactness but also to some of his other basic series. Table 13 illustrates the scope of stridency for Jakobson and Trubetzkoy, respectively.

A comparison between the two classifications shows that stridency, as applied to the labials, is identical for Jakobson and Trubetzkoy, except that Trubetzkoy also accommodated the affricate /p̌/ as strident in opposition to /m/.

Digressing to Chomsky and Halle (1968), the distinction between labials and labiodentals is fitted here into the category +/– distributed. Chomsky and Halle, however, pointed out that "the fact that there are other feature distinctions between these two classes of sounds which makes this distinction in length of stricture somewhat peripheral, though no less real" (1968, p. 314). For the physical correlate of +/– distributed, see above, p. 89.

In reference to the dentals and palatals, although Trubetzkoy had spoken of the possible binarity between the apical and sibilant series, he did not make explicit by what feature such a relationship would be handled. He used the stridency feature to differentiate between the sibilants. This differs from Jakobson's use of the feature, which treated the distinction between the sibilants by gravity, leaving stridency to distinguish the dentals and the palatals from their respective sibilant opposites. Thus, dental /θ/ is distinguished from the sibilant /s/ by the opposition mellow/ strident.

With respect to the gutturals, that is, the opposition between velars and uvulars in terms of stridency, Chomsky and Halle pointed out that "the earlier framework [Jakobsonian] made it impossible in principle to distinguish velar from uvular or pharyngeal consonants by means of their points of articulation," and "that such distinction had to be made by use of some subsidiary feature such as stridency" (p. 308). They called attention to the fact that there were languages in which "velar and uvular consonants do not differ in any such feature, and could therefore not be accounted for" (1968, p. 308). Chomsky and Halle analyzed the different points of articulation (velar, uvular, pharyngeal) by a combination of the features high, low, back, anterior, and coronal.

Comparing the three feature systems, it would seem that Trubetzkoy's is a middle road between Jakobson and Chomsky-Halle with respect to the latter classes referred to. He established an independent class of laryngeals, which was then also split by the stridency feature.

The Trubetzkoyan division of the guttural series into prevelar and postvelar consonants appears to correspond to the Jakobsonian division of the guttrual consonants into velars and uvulars by the stridency feature.

In reference to the third point above, the distinction between stops and affricates had not been specifically listed by Trubetzkoy as one of stridency. However, in the labial series affricates were contrasted with the nasals by the feature stridency.

In *Observations* Jakobson opposed the German affricates /pf/ and /t͡s/ to the stops /p/ and /t/ as strident versus mellow. Not specifically discussed was the relationship between simple stops, affricates, and constrictives, as in /p-pf-f/ and /t-t͡s-s/, which is found in Standard German. This relationship caused a dilemma since both the opposition of /p/ to /f/ and /p/ to /pf/, according to Jakobson's own representations, had to be considered as mellow versus strident (1938, p. 277).

In *Preliminaries* two solutions were offered to this problem. One relied on a single ternary opposition, the other on two binary oppositions. According to the first solution, the distinction between /p-p̌(=pf)-f/ was analyzed in terms of the opposition of optimal constrictive versus optimal stop. Thus:

I.	/f/	/p/	/p̌/
Optimal constrictive	+	−	±

Optimal here implied the coalescence of two features having the same plus or minus value. Optimal constrictive thus has the features + strident, + constrictive (continuant), and optimal stop has the features − strident, − constrictive.

In terms of a binary solution, and using the features of constrictiveness (continuance) and stridency separately, the three way contrast was analyzed as follows:

II.	/f/	/p/	/p̌/
Constrictiveness	+	−	−
Stridency	+	−	+

Implicit in the second solution was that the closure of /p̌/ was considered primary in contrast to the subsequent constriction. Jakobson favored a binary solution with two features since "it is preferable to deal with simple two-choice situations" (Jakobson, Fant, and Halle, 1952, p. 25).

As indicated above, Trubetzkoy used the stridency feature in slightly different contrasts. In contrast to *Preliminaries,* where /p-p̌-f/ are opposed, he did not oppose /p̌/ to /p/ by stridency. Instead he contrasted /p̌/ to /m/ (and so presumably also /t͡s/ to /n/ instead of to /t/) by the feature strident/mellow.

As already noted in conjunction with the dentals and palatals, stridency could take on a gradual character in the Trubetzkoyan classification. This was the case in the ternary opposition /s-ŝ-š/ found in Low Sorbian (a West Slavic language) and Kabardian (a language spoken in the North West Caucasus) (1939/1969, p. 129). The stridency feature there had to be considered as actually ternary in contrast to the above examples of *Preliminaries* carrying the notation ±, where the feature optimal constrictiveness had actually consisted of two collapsed or fused features.

The example of the laryngeal listed in Table 13 is a further Trubetzkoyan distinction involving stridency; it was not made by Jakobson. Trubetzkoy did not specifically include the liquids into the opposition of stridency as Jakobson did in *Preliminaries.*

In their discussion of stridency, which opposed the affricates to the stops as strident versus mellow, Chomsky and Halle (1968, p. 321ff.) pointed out that this treatment did not allow for the existence of nonstrident affricates. They maintained that such a class actually exists (Chippewa, a North American Indian language, is said to have contrasting dental strident and nonstrident affricates) and therefore proposed to treat the distinction between stops and affricates by a *release* feature. This feature contrasts stops with "instantaneous release" to stops with "delayed release." The feature of stridency then is available to distinguish between strident and nonstrident affricates.[73]

From what has been said, it appears that stridency is losing its grounds as a feature, being replaced by or realigned with various others, and may be doomed to disappear altogether. The reason for this is partially that the existence of a finer distinction has been discovered. Furthermore, the disparity in the phonological oppositions analyzed by this feature, which included the oppositions between stops and affricates, velars and uvulars, labials and labiodentals, would constitute an uneasy basis for any theory claiming to have articulatory and/or acoustic correlates. In some ways the stridency feature has also become obsolete within the present theory. Oppositions previously accommodated by stridency in the Chomsky-Halle framework could also be handled by other features which constituted innovations in the present framework (see above, p. 87 ff.).[74]

Trubetzkoy did not handle all the divisions in the basic series with the stridency feature. The following divisions remained:

> The split of the apical series:
> Alveolar (postdental)
> Retroflex
>
> Alveolar
> Interdental
>
> Dental
> Dental-palatal[75]
>
> The split of the guttural series:[75]
> Velar
> Labiovelar
>
> Velar
> Palatal

Trubetzkoy opposed the above series to each other by the opposition flat/plain. In a way it is curious to note that, at least in part, Trubetzkoy's physical correlate for this opposition comes close to the correlates used by Jakobson in *Observations* for the opposition grave/acute. Jakobson's physical correlate for the grave consonants was "a long and undivided resonator" as compared to the acute consonants, where "the tongue divides the oral cavity into two" short resonator compartments" (1938/1962, p. 274). In *Grundzüge* the difference between flat/plain was also defined as one essentially related to the difference in the length of the oral resonator. As Jakobson did for the opposition grave/acute, Trubetzkoy acoustically likened the difference between the opposition flat/plain to the lowering and heightening of timbre for the split in the guttural series. Trubetzkoy had contrasted the retroflexes and the apicals as sounds with a flat timbre (*mit hohem Klang*) to sounds with a plain timbre (*flachem Klang*). This acoustically impressionistic distinction was then also transferred to the opposition between velars and labiovelars. Trubetzkoy noted that it was not quite as easy to make this distinction so clearly for the opposition between dentals and palatals, velars and palatals, and alveolars and interdentals. He nevertheless used the flatness feature for these oppositions as well.

The opposition flat/plain had not yet appeared in *Observations,* where labiovelars and retroflexes had been left unanalyzed. In *Preliminaries,* Jakobson apparently followed Trubetzkoy's lead and accommodated these classes into his system by the use of the flatness feature. In *Grundzüge* the physical correlate of the flatness feature was related to differences in the length of the anterior resonator. For the retroflexes, the physical correlates were seen in terms of a modification in volume and shape of the two resonating cavities (in front and back of position of articulation). On the other hand, the flatness feature in *Preliminaries* related to "orifice variation." The physical correlate was stated in terms of a "reduction of the lip orifice (rounding) with a concomitant increase in the length of the lip constriction" (Jakobson, Fant, and Halle, 1952, p. 31). Jakobson also included rounding in vowels in his flatness feature; Trubetzkoy did not. Trubetzkoy also excluded pharyngeals, in contrast to Jakobson, who included pharyngeals under the flatness feature, based on the rationale that "instead of the front orifice of the mouth cavity, the pharyngeal tract, in its turn, may be contracted with a similar effect of flattening" (Jakobson, Fant, and Halle, 1952, p. 31). But with respect to the retroflexes, "both the contraction of the pharynx and the elongation of the resonating cavity take place in producing emphatic as well as retroflex consonants, but for the former the first process, and for the latter the second one seems to be of greater pertinence" (Jakobson, Fant, and Halle, 1952, p. 34) In the case of the retroflex consonants the physical correlates of Trubetzkoy and Jakobson for flatness were thus equivalent.

For Jakobson the flatness feature also applied to liquids and glides (Jakobson, Fant, and Halle, 1952, p. 34) and included the glottal stop and /h/. Neither of these is considered in the class of liquids and glides by Trubetzkoy.[76]

The flatness feature distinguished for Trubetzkoy between velars and palatals and between dentals and palatals (under conditions detailed earlier). Jakobson handled these with the opposition grave/acute and compact/diffuse, respectively.

Trubetzkoy cited examples of gradual relationships for the features stridency and flatness. He maintained that in languages which had a palatal series in addition to retroflex and plain apicals, or alveolars and interdentals, such an opposition could be considered as a ternary one of flatness. The ternary character would become even clearer when supported by evidence of neutralization between the palatal and one of the apical series. Trubetzkoy maintained that it was also possible to interpret the three respective classes of phonemes as three different degrees of raising or lowering the tip of the tongue, since this was relevant for the apicals. This physical correlate served as a rationale for interpreting the three classes of sounds as three-way split in the apical series that could be accommodated by the flatness feature.

In addition to flat/plain, Jakobson also set up the feature sharp/plain, in which the "oral cavity is reduced by raising a part of the tongue against the palate" (Jakobson, Fant, and Halle, 1952, p. 31). This resulted in palatalization. The additional feature of sharpness in effect constituted a split in the earlier flatness feature. The original ternary character of flatness is evidenced from the physical description for the two features. The opposition flat/plain "opposes narrowed slit phonemes to wider slit phonemes" and the opposition plain/sharp "opposes narrower slit phonemes to widened slit phonemes" (Jakobson and Halle, 1956, p. 31). But while the original ternary distinction in *Grundzüge* also included the palatals, the division in *Preliminaries* only appears to comprise secondary articulation—in other words, palatalization.

Secondary Series: Relationship Between Primary and Secondary Articulation   In addition to the basic series and the related series, Trubetzkoy posited several secondary series which stood in a relation of privative opposition to each other, representing a split in the basic and the related series. Accordingly, the opposition relationships discussed below were represented by the three types of series: basic, related, and secondary:[77]

1. *Basic series:* Oppositions in the basic series could be defined as those in which the contrastive pair stood in a multilateral heterogenous opposition relationship to each other. Each of

the basic series stands in a relation of multilateral opposition to the other basic series (see above, p. 109).

2. *Related series:* Oppositions in the related series could be defined as those which stood in an equipollent bilateral opposition relationship to each other. (If a related series was the result of a reinterpretation of a basic series, the contrastive pairs stood in a relationship of privative, bilateral (neutralizable) opposition to each other.)

3. *Secondary series:* Oppositions in the secondary series could be defined as those which stood in a privative opposition relationship to each other and represent a split into two series each of the basic and related series.

From Figure 7 it seems clear that the opposition relationships within the secondary series are the most translucent since they are based on the presence versus the absence of a feature (hence privative). The secondary series in this classification consisted of sound classes in which the articulatory organs perform a secondary function not directly associated with their primary articulatory task. According to Trubetzkoy, this could have one of two effects: the resultant sounds either had a kind of "vocalic timbre" (or coloration) or they were click sounds.

Trubetzkoy set up several such secondary series. Given in terms of correlations, these were:

1. Labialization
2. Labiovelarization
3. Palatalization
4. Emphatic palatalization
5. Full gutturalization
6. Emphatic velarization
7. Retroflexion
8. Click

Comparing the Trubetzkoyan with the subsequent classification by Jakobson, Fant, and Halle in *Preliminaries,* it should be pointed out that Jakobson did not make the distinction in features between primary and secondary articulation. However, the following five observations can be made regarding the accommodations of these secondary series in their classification.

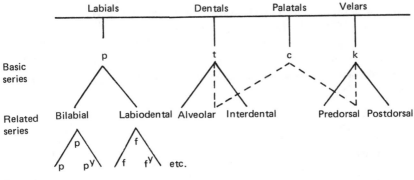

Figure 7. Examples of opposition relationships in the three series, basic, related, and secondary. (Partial representation.)

First, the Trubetzkoyan correlation of emphatic velarization appears under the name "pharyngealization" in *Preliminaries* and is part of the opposition flat/plain.

Second, the correlation of labiovelarization was interpreted by Trubetzkoy as a composite of the correlations of labialization and of full gutturalization. This interpretation was not explicitly given in *Preliminaries,* where labiovelarization is subsumed under the opposition flat/plain.

Third, in *Preliminaries,* Jakobson, Fant, and Halle reinterpreted the above correlations of emphatic velarization (pharyngealization), labialization, full gutturalization, labiovelarization, and retroflexion in terms of the opposition flat/plain. In substituting one feature for all of these correlations, Jakobson and his co-workers appeared to have been governed by the principles of economy and of complementary distribution. The principle of complementary distribution is here applied across languages. These correlations tend to occur mutually exclusively in one language (but see below). Jakobson also included the feature vowel rounding in the flatness feature.

Fourth, Jakobson's opposition sharp/plain substituted for the Trubetzkoyan correlation of palatalization.

Fifth, it is not clear from *Preliminaries* and *Fundamentals* whether the correlation of emphatic palatalization was to be considered a variation of palatalization that could be included in the opposition sharp/plain or whether it was to be considered a variation of velarization and therefore could belong to the opposition flat/plain. The latter appears to be the case. According to Trubetzkoy, the correlation of emphatic palatalization is found in the languages of the Eastern Caucasus, such as Chechen, Ingush, and Bats. The articulatory, physical correlates of emphatic palatalization were described as:

> . . . a reduction of the resonator orifice . . . produced mainly by an upward shift of the larynx by which the body of the tongue is also moved toward the front. The special position of the larynx in the production of emphatic-palatalized consonants produces a specific "hoarse" fricative noise which extends to the neighboring vowels as well. (Trubetzkoy, 1939/1969, p. 131)

The physical correlates for the opposition flat/plain in *Preliminaries* were described as follows (see also above, p. 117):

> Flattening is chiefly generated by a reduction of the lip orifice (rounding) with a concomitant increase in the length of the lip constriction. Hence . . . orifice variation. (Jakobson, Fant, and Halle, 1952, p. 31)

And:

> Instead of the front orifice of the mouth cavity, the pharyngeal tract in its turn may be contracted with a similar flattening. (ibid.)

In *Fundamentals* the opposition was described as follows:

> Flat (narrowed slit) phonemes in contradistinction with the latter [wider slit] phonemes are produced with a decreased back or front orifice of the mouth resonator. (Jakobson and Halle, 1956, p. 31)

The physical correlates for the opposition sharp/plain as given in *Preliminaries* were described in the following way:

> To effect this feature, the oral cavity is reduced by raising a part of the tongue against the palate. This adjustment, called palatalization, is made simultaneously with the main articulation of a given consonant and is linked with a greater dilation of the pharyngeal pass in comparison with the corresponding plain consonant. (Jakobson, Fant, and Halle, 1952, p. 31)

This opposition was described in *Fundamentals:*

> . . . the sharp (widened slit) v. plain (narrower slit) phonemes exhibit a dilated pharyngeal pass, i.e., a widened back orifice of the mouth resonator. A concomitant palatalization restricts and compartments the mouth cavity. (Jakobson and Halle, 1956, p. 31)

According to Jakobson (personal communication) both Trubetzkoy and he covered approximately the same ground with respect to the flatness feature. In *Preliminaries* and *Fundamentals*, however, the emphasis seem to be on secondary articulation with respect to flatness, while this was not the case in *Grundzüge*. As pointed out above, *Grundzüge* did not include a sharpness feature; this was first mentioned in *Preliminaries*. The flatness feature of *Grundzüge* could take on a gradual ternary character. According to Jakobson, sharpness was the result of a split of the flat/plain opposition which, however, only covered secondary articulation (palatalization). Primary articulations, that is, the palatals, were already covered by compactness and gravity in the Jakobsonian classification. This was not the case in the Trubetzkoyan classification, where the palatals were considered either a basic or a related series in connection with the flatness feature.

It seems that what Trubetzkoy called "full gutturalization" can be equated with the subsequent notion of "extreme velarization" in Chomsky and Halle (1968). In *Grundzüge* the articulatory correlates for the feature of full gutturalization consisted of:

> . . . raising the dorsum of the tongue against the soft palate. The tongue can be raised high enough so as to practically form a velar closure (example Zezuru dialect of Shona). Or it may be raised somewhat lower so that it result only in a velar stricture. (1939/1969, p. 137)[78]

Velarization and labiovelarization, according to Trubetzkoy, were not mutually exclusive (1939/1969, p. 138). That Jakobson appeared to consider them so within a language is evident from the fact that he included both of them in the opposition flat/plain. (The examples given by Trubetzkoy were from the Eastern and Central Shona dialects: /p͡k, c͡k, t͡kw, c͡kw/.)

Finally, Trubetzkoy also interpreted the click correlation as a secondary series. Based on the fact that clicks are characterized by two closures, Jakobson interpreted these as successive in *Preliminaries*. He considered the clicks as consonant clusters, a solution that must have seemed somewhat counterintuitive from the start. The relation of Trubetzkoy's conception of clicks to that of Jakobson is discussed further below.

In summary, these secondary series, with the exception of the click correlation, were considered in the Jakobsonian classification as belonging to the oppositions flat/plain and sharp/plain. As noted earlier, Trubetzkoy had established the opposition flat/plain to account for some opposition relationships between his basic and related series. The opposition sharp/plain had not yet existed within the Trubetzkoyan framework.

This leads to the following questions, which are examined below: What was the relationship between the secondary series and the basic and related series within the Trubetzkoyan classification? How did the Trubetzkoyan classification, as it relates to these three series, compare to that of Jakobson and to the new feature classification by Chomsky and Halle?

Relationship Between the Secondary Series and the Basic and Related Series and Between These and Jakobson's Classification   Although Trubetzkoy had not yet formalized explicit rules to that effect, he appeared to have based his classification on several considerations which can be summarized as follows from his exposition in *Grundzüge* (1939/1969, p. 132ff.). One and the same feature could serve to cover several distinctions in those cases where a language has both a secondary series and a basic or related series and where: 1) the superimposed supplementary articulation of the secondary series also constituted the primary articulation in the basic or related series, and 2) the respective basic or related series and the secondary series were also mutually exclusive.

This could occur in the case of the basic series of the palatals and the secondary one of palatalization. The palatals were then considered either as palatalized apicals or as palatalized gutturals. The opposition between palatals and apicals, or palatals and gutturals, was then under certain circumstances considered as one of flat/plain. The opposition between labiovelars and velars, and retroflexes and apicals, was also considered as one of flat/ plain:

> The palatal series cannot exist as an autonomous series of localiza-
> tion in languages with simple palatalization, because it is inevita-
> bly interpreted as "palatalized apical" or "palatalized guttural."
> (Trubetzkoy, 1939/1969, p. 131)

According to Trubetzkoy, the same relationship held for the secondary series of emphatic palatalization and a basic pharyngeal series, the latter being interpreted as palatalized laryngeals. The relationship of mutual exclusion between primary and secondary articulation did not hold true for the labial series and labialization, which could co-occur (for example, Burmese /p, p°/).

It is not quite clear from *Grundzüge* which feature should be used to express this complementary relationship between the basic and secondary series. For example, should the distinction between palatalization and the palatals be expressed in terms of palatalization or flatness, which had already been used for primary articulation?

An important difference between Trubetzkoy and Jakobson with respect to the above is that Trubetzkoy recognized certain specific relationships of articulatory relatedness and mutual exclusion between his secondary series and his basic or related series (for example, palatalization and palatals), but he also used these as principles for classification. This was not always true for Jakobson. For example, the relationship between palatals and palatalization and velars and velarization in Jakobson's classification was obscured by the use of two distinct features, gravity (or compactness, respectively), and flatness, (or sharpness, respectively). However, the use of different features by Jakobson may be interpreted as indicative of the fact that in the one case the articulatory correlates are primary and in the other they are mainly secondary (at least with respect to the consonants). But such a differentiation between primary and secondary articulation was not always made by means of different features. For example, in *Mufaxxama* (1957, p. 519), Jakobson wrote with respect to the Arabic /ayn/:

> /ayn/ is merely the *flat feature*, while the pharyngealized buccals, sometimes labeled "/ayn/" phonemes, *superimpose flatness upon a bundle of other features*. (1957, p. 519; emphasis added)

Relatedness between primary and secondary articulation was recognized by Jakobson here, although mutual exclusion was not specifically mentioned. Notable in this quotation is that within the Jakobsonian framework the phoneme /ayn/ was accorded less of a feature status than the other phonemes that have pharyngealization superimposed.[79]

McCawley, in *Le role d'un système des traits phonologiques dan une théorie du langage* (1967), pointed out that rounding and pharyngealization were not always mutually exclusive. In discussing the feature specification in the phonological component, McCawley called attention to the fact that in Arabic both rounding and pharyngealization are present. In a theory in which the phonological component would operate in terms of the opposition flat/plain, and where "rounding" and "pharyngealization" only played a role in the interpretative rules of features, the following rule would have to be included in the phonological component:

$$[+\text{Syllabic}] \rightarrow [+\text{Flat}] \bigg/ \left\{ \begin{array}{l} \underline{\hspace{3cm}} \quad \left[\begin{array}{l} +\text{Flat} \\ -\text{Syllabic} \end{array} \right] \\[2ex] \left[\begin{array}{l} +\text{Flat} \\ -\text{Syllabic} \end{array} \right] \quad \underline{\hspace{3cm}} \end{array} \right.$$

The interpretive rules would then have to specify that the feature flat is to be interpreted as pharyngealized for consonants or for front or open vowels, as rounded when it refers to close back vowels, and as "rounded" and "pharyngealized" when it refers to close back vowels adjacent to a flat consonant.

From a classical Jakobsonian viewpoint it is doubtful whether the above problem would ever have arisen, for mutually exclusive meant distinctively so. The phonological system of Arabic contains three vowels of the type /i, u, a/. In all likelihood flatness in the vowel /u/ would have been considered redundant by Jakobson, since he considered gravity primary. Such a position was in fact reflected by the Arabic vowel system which appeared in *Preliminaries* (p. 34). The reinterpreting of flatness for vowels as distinctive would have been possible, of course, but not necessary. It hinged on the interpretation of the following statement in *Preliminaries*:

> If there is only one tonality feature in the vowels of a given language, then it may be lumped with the primary (or only) tonality feature of the consonants. (Jakobson, Fant, and Halle, 1952, p. 33)

Since Arabic has both the gravity and the flatness features for consonants (Trubetzkoy, 1939/1969 p. 132), the question thus would be which of the features is primary.

Relationship Between the Trubetzkoyan Classification and the Classification of Chomsky and Halle   The above features are related to the phonological framework expanded in *The Sound Pattern of English* in several ways. Chomsky and Halle, in their feature classification, reworked and replaced the features flat/plain and sharp/plain for a number of reasons.

First, they noted that the use of these features obscures the relationship between the palatals, velars, and pharyngeals on the one hand, and the above three types of secondary articulation on the other. It also obscures the vowel-like coloration of the secondary series. Chomsky and Halle stated with respect to the secondary articulation:

> The subsidiary articulation consists in the superimposition of vowel-like articulations on the basic consonantal articulation. (1968, p. 305)

Trubetzkoy had also expressed such a vowel-like effect when he wrote:

> The acoustic result of the secondary series is either a specific coloration, that is, a kind of vocalic timbre [or a click sound]. (1939/1969, p. 129)

In the new framework of *Sound Pattern* both the primary and the secondary articulations were handled by a combination of the features high, low, and back. These features also covered the vowels implicated in the acoustic impression of the secondary series.

Formalizing the impression that palatalization is i-like, velarization i-like, pharyngealization a-like, Chomsky and Halle considered palatalized consonants as +high, −back, velarized consonants as +high, +back, and pharyngealized consonants as +low, +back.

In the Jakobsonian framework the feature sharpness had only applied to consonants and the parallel between vowels and consonants for that feature had thus been lost.

The above concordances between primary and secondary articulation in vowels is shown in Table 14.

Trubetzkoy had pointed out the similarities between specific vowels and the earlier noted secondary articulations in consonants. However, he did not expressly relate the features for the consonants to the specific ones used for the vowels. The

Table 14. Chomsky-Halle classification of primary and secondary articulation in consonants and vowels using the features high, back, and low

Feature	Palatals, palatalization; /i/	Velars, velarization; /ɨ/	Pharyngeals, pharyngealization; /a/
High	+	+	−
Back	−	+	+
Low	−	−	+

Chomsky-Halle classification in Table 14, therefore, represents an improvement over the Jakobsonian classification and in some ways comes closer to the earlier Trubetzkoyan classification expressing the relationship between the basic and the secondary series, and the secondary series and the vowels.

The second reason Chomsky and Halle reclassified the features flat/plain and sharp/plain was that they wanted to distinguish secondary articulation as it related to palatalization (sharpness), velarization, and pharyngealization (flatness), from that of labialization. As mentioned earlier, labialization or rounding in the Jakobsonian framework had been covered by the flatness feature, as had retroflexion. In the new Chomsky-Halle framework, labialization was handled by the feature rounding. Retroflexion and retroflexes were covered by the feature $+/-$ distributed. Only the latter were mentioned as covered by that feature in *Sound Pattern*. It may be assumed, however, that Chomsky and Halle also wished to include retroflexion in the feature $+/-$ distributed, since retroflexion of consonants or retroflex consonants only appear to be alternative ways of expression. A superimposed feature of retroflexion can only be conceived of with respect to the vowels, while retroflexion (in consonants) can be interpreted as a primary or a secondary articulatory feature.

Chomsky and Halle had valid reasons for reanalyzing the flatness and sharpness features in terms of high, low, and back, namely, as noted earlier, to cover velarization, pharyngealization, and palatalization. They wanted to bring out the parallels between primary and secondary articulation in consonants and in vowels. However, some of their factual assumptions associated with such a reanalysis were incorrect. In *Sound Pattern,* following a justification for replacing the feature of diffuseness by high/nonhigh for vowels and by anterior/nonanterior for consonants, they said:

> A further consequence . . . [in the Jakobsonian framework] was the need to characterize palatalization, velarization, and pharyngealization by means of independent features. *This in turn failed to explain why these subsidiary articulations are not found with consonants that are formed with the body of the tongue,* i.e., consonants that are non-coronal and non-anterior in the present framework. (1968, p. 307; emphasis added)

Chomsky and Halle point out that:

> In the former framework this was a mere accident, in the revised framework this is structurally motivated. It is worthy to note that rounding (labialization) which is a subsidiary articulation, is not subject to similar restrictions. All classes of consonants, including labials, may be rounded. (1968, p. 307)

With respect to the above, two points may be underscored. First, the distinction of labialization from the above three types of secondary articulation, which had been absent in the Jakobsonian classification, was based on the distributional variable that labials and labialization were not mutually exclusive. This distinction had already been referred to by Trubetzkoy.

Second, however, segregating the above three types of secondary articulation from labialization as an explanation of why these subsidiary articulations were not found with consonants formed with the body of the tongue, that is, with consonants that are noncoronal and nonanterior, was obviously based on incorrect and incomplete factual representation and represented an overgeneralization.

Chomsky and Halle themselves vitiated the statement quoted above when they said, in discussing the number of possible categories of a phonological matrix:

> Thus to take just one of innumerable examples, in Modern Hebrew the feature of pharyngealization is phonetically lost in stops, but it must still be marked in lexical matrices to prevent post-vocalic spirantization in what is historically an emphatic /k/ for example. Thus we have [kavar] [lixbor] contrasting with [kavar] [likbor], *and we may account for the contrast by representing the former with a non-pharyngealized [k] and the latter with a pharyngealized [k]*. (1968, p. 170, fn. 7; emphasis added)

It seems that what Chomsky and Halle meant to express was that for the labials and labialization the principle of complementary distribution does not apply with respect to primary and secondary articulation in the same segment, but in each of the other three cases it does. Accordingly, what should have been expressed was the following series of rules:

1. Velarization does not occur with velars
2. Palatalization does not occur with palatals
3. Pharyngealization does not occur with pharyngeals
4. Labialization does co-occur with labials

Naturally their above overgeneralization is not explanatory of this fact. The inaccuracy of this generalization also collapses the cleverly conceived alternation between primary and secondary articulation in feature representation.

With respect to retroflexes and retroflexion, which were not included in the Chomsky-Halle generalization, it is not quite possible to make such a neat distinction. As mentioned earlier, it is hardly possible to differentiate between, on the one hand, a retroflex point of articulation which would be primary and, on the other, a secondary feature of retroflexion—at least not as far as the consonants are concerned. Here primary and secondary articulation are mutually exclusive with respect to all consonants.

In reference to the clicks, Trubetzkoy had considered important a basic frontal closure in addition to a supplemental closure, and the resultant modification of the shape of the tongue, and "hence the configuration of the entire oral resonating cavity" (1939/1969a, p. 135 ff.). Chomsky and Halle credited Trubetzkoy for recognizing this. They considered click consonants instances of extreme velarization. They further posited a suction feature for the clicks:

> We differ from Trubetzkoy, however, in postulating a special feature (suction) to account for the peculiar release of these secondary constrictions.

It may be added that Trubetzkoy had not neglected the suction element, but he did not consider it distinctive:

> The pressure of two closures, of which one must be velar and the other somewhere in the anterior part of the oral cavity, is part of the nature of click sounds. A suction act rarifies the air between the two closures, outside air rushes into the airstarved space. But immediately thereafter, the posterior velar closure is released. (1939/1969, p. 136)

But:

> If one compares the clicks and the fully gutturalized (or labiovelarized) consonants, one arrives at the conclusion that the difference is only phonetic, not phonological. The suction element which, at first glance, seems to be so characteristic of clicks, is only a special way of releasing the anterior oral closure. For the position of the click sounds in the phonemic system it is much less important than the presence of the velar "supplemental closure." But the latter is also present in the pure gutturalized and labiovelarized consonants (of Zezuru and the other dialects of Eastern and Central Shona), though perhaps not in quite as energetic a form. (1939/1969, p. 136)

A difference between Chomsky-Halle and Trubetzkoy with respect to the click sounds is that for Trubetzkoy velar closure was always supplemental. In contrast, based on data from African languages, such as Kpelle, Chomsky and Halle claimed that this is not always the case. For them, primacy of velar closure was established on the basis of assimilation evidence, for example, nasals → [+ back] in the environment of labiovelars and velars.

Labials and Labialization in Consonants and Rounding in Vowels Chomsky and Halle sought to express the relatedness found to hold between several aspects of the sound spectrum by revamping the feature system and establishing the features high, back, and low. These features applied to vowels as well as to consonants for both primary and secondary articulation.

It would also be desirable for their "renovated" feature classification to express the relations holding between the labials, labialization, and rounding in vowels. Their new classification does this only to an extent: rounding covers labialization in consonants and rounding in vowels.

As mentioned earlier, even though Trubetzkoy classified vowels and consonants separately, he recognized the relationship between labialization in consonants and rounding in vowels. His secondary series, in which "the vocal organs perform a secondary task . . . not involved directly in the basic task" were described acoustically as a "kind of vocalic timbre" (or alternatively, as click sounds) (1939/1969, p. 129). The critical element in labialization in consonants and rounding in vowels was lip participation.

Relatedness between the labials and labialization in consonants was evident from the labels for these categories themselves as well as from a discussion of examples involved. (see further below).

To provide an explanation for the universality of the three basic series, labials, apicals, and gutturals, Trubetzkoy wrote:

> This [their universality] certainly cannot be an accident. It must have some basis in the makeup of these three series. It is probably easiest to seek an explanation in the fact that the *lips*, the tip of the tongue, and the dorsum of the tongue are movable organs that are best suited for obstructing the oral cavity. *Thus for the labials, the bringing together of the lips is relevant* . . . (1939/1969, p. 123; emphasis added)

Rounding in vowels Trubetzkoy also had described in terms of lip participation (1939/1969, p. 97 ff.).

The relationship between the various types of lip participation, that is of rounding in vowels and of primary and secondary articulation in consonants was illustrated by Trubetzkoy by the example below. Discussing the three-vowel system of Adyghe (a language of the North West Caucasus), he provided the following distributional information:

> . . . the maximally close ə . . . is realized as u in the neighborhood of *labialized velars,* as ü between *two labials,* and after *labialized sibilants,* as ɯ after non-labialized back velars, as i after palatals, and in all other positions as a close indeterminate vowel ə; mid open e . . . is realized after *labialized velars* as o, after *labialized sibilants* and between *labials* as ö, after laryngeals and non-labialized back velars as a, in the remaining positions as e or as indeterminate open vowel ë; and the maximally open a which is realized between two *labials* as slightly *rounded,* between two palatals as ä, and elsewhere as a long ä. (1939/1969, p. 97; emphasis added)

The way in which the relationship between vowel articulation and primary and secondary consonant articulation was expressed in the Jakobsonian classification deserves attention.

As already pointed out, the Jakobsonian classification partially observed the close relationship between primary and secondary articulation. The relationship was obscured for the labials and labialization, velars and velarization, and palatals and palatalization. In the case of the pharyngeals and pharyngealization, and the retroflexes and retroflexion, this had not been the case. (Neither had it been the case with respect to labiovelars and labiovelarization.) The feature flatness had been used to cover secondary and primary articulation.

For labialization in consonants and rounding in vowels, relatedness had been expressed by the shared use of the flatness feature. The rest of the pertinent vowel features were the same as those used for the primary articulation of consonants (gravity and compactness).

Jakobson, however, distinguished between primary and secondary articulation to some extent. He did so by using different features and by lumping secondary articulation together on the basis of the distributional criterion of mutual exclusion. Palatalization had been segregated from the other secondary features at least partially, because it could co-occur with labialization and thus would have vitiated the principle of mutual exclusion vis-à-vis the other secondary features. (Examples for the co-occurrence of palatalization and labialization given by Trubetzkoy included

Ubyk and Dungan Chinese (1969/1969, p. 132).) In summary, then, with the exception of the rounding in vowels, primary and secondary articulation were treated fairly separately in the Jakobsonian classification.

Chomsky and Halle (1968) used the feature rounding to cover rounding in vowels and labialization in consonants. They thus mirrored the relationship presented in the Jakobsonian classification, where the flatness feature was used for rounding in vowels and for labialization. In the Chomsky-Halle classification rounded sounds "are produced with a narrowing of the lip orifice; non-rounded sounds are produced without such narrowing" (1968, p. 309). For Jakobson, flattening was chiefly generated by "the reduction of the lip orifice with a concomitant increase in the length of the lip constriction . . ." (Jakobson, Fant, and Halle, 1952, p. 31; see also above, p. 122).

Chomsky and Halle claimed that the degree of rounding was always determinable from other features. They distinguished phonetically between at least three different degrees of rounding for consonants. They noted that in most languages "an extreme degree of rounding (i.e., total lip closure) was a feature of the velars" (1968, p. 311). Following Ladefoged (1964, p. 47), they cited Temme, an African language, as an example of the phonetic, feature-dependent distinction between a moderate and extreme degree of rounding. In Temme, "a voiceless plosive with a moderate degree of rounding [kʷ] is paired with a voiced plosive with extreme rounding [gᵇ]."[80]

It seems that "extreme rounding" in the above case was analogous to a secondary labial stop, especially if we are to believe the validity of the phonetic symbols used in the description. However, Chomsky and Halle did not characterize labials in terms of rounding but in terms of +anterior, −coronal, −high, −low, −back (1968, p. 307).

The glides, as related to the vowels, also carry the feature of rounding phonetically. According to Chomsky and Halle:

French distinguishes three glides phonetically: non-round, non-back [y] as in *les yeux* 'the eyes,' round, back [w] as in *les oiseaux* 'the birds,' and round, non-back [ẅ] as in *tuer* 'to kill.' (1968, p. 309)

The glides, as listed, were distinguished from each other by the features high, low, and back (in addition to the features anterior and coronal).

Thus, a parallel was established between the palatals, palatalization, and the /y/ glide. However, a parallel between the labials, labialization, and /w/ is lacking. Instead there is a parallel in features between velarization and the /w/. Both were classified in terms of +high, −low, +back, as well as −anterior and −coronal. /w/ contains both a velar and a labial element, though intuitively it would seem that rounding is more prominent than velarity. However, within the Chomsky-Halle framework it was not possible to bring out both the relationship of /w/ to the velars and velarization and to labials and labialization. It seems that a parallel between /w/, the labials, and labialization should be expressed in their feature system (especially in the light of their example of the various degrees of rounding which had phonetically been represented by [w] and [b]). However, the Chomsky-Halle characterization of /w/ and the labials differ considerably, as shown in Table 15.

It would appear that a re-examination of the Chomsky-Halle feature system is warranted with respect to this point. However, if under the existing system the labials were to be specified in terms of rounding, a different type of problem would arise: it may become necessary to use the feature rounding twice for the same segment. There may be instances in which rounding would have to be specified as primary for labials; and in view of the existence of labialized labials, rounding would also have to be specified for secondary articulation. However, even without such a problem, specifying the relationship of primary and secondary articulation formally would still be fraught with difficulties.

In discussing the feature specification for labiovelars, Chomsky and Halle considered two alternatives: the labiovelars could be represented as velarized labials or as labialized velars:

1. Velarized labial:
   + Anterior
   − Coronal
   + Back
   + High

2. Labialized velars:
   − Anterior
   − Coronal
   + Back
   + High
   + Round

The parallel between the labials and labialization is, of course, lost here, since labiality is expressed by + anterior, − coronal, in

Table 15.   Chomsky-Halle characterization of labials,
/w/, and velars

	Anterior	Coronal	High	Low	Back
Labials	+	−	−	−	−
Glide /w/	−	−	+	−	+
Velars	−	−	+	−	+

contrast to labialization, which was expressed by +rounding.
Representing labiovelars as labialized velars also necessitated an
additional feature as compared to their representation as velarized labials. However, both solutions intuitively should have
the same number of features.

The two matrices also represented different facts. In the first
matrix, velarized labials, the −high and −back of the primary
articulation appeared to be redundant in the environment of
+anterior, −coronal, and in the environment of the secondary
articulation +back, +high. They were thus left out. The feature
low is specified as a minus for velars and labials (and hence also
for velarized labials).

With respect to labialized velars, the representation was
specified as −anterior, −coronal. Although −low was dropped,
+high and +back were retained. The feature rounding was also
added. It seems that the relationship which should have been
expressed with respect to velarized labials and labialized velars is
the following:

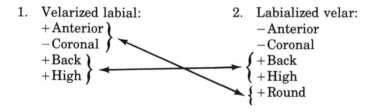

1. Velarized labial:
    +Anterior
    −Coronal
    +Back
    +High

2. Labialized velar:
    −Anterior
    −Coronal
    +Back
    +High
    +Round

Lip participation in the specification of the velarized labial belonged to primary articulation while lip participation in the

specification of the labialized velar belonged to secondary articulation. Conversely, the same held true for velarity.

As mentioned earlier, if the feature rounding were to include the labials, the resultant problem would be that in some instances rounding would have to be specified twice, once for primary and once for secondary articulation. This is so because the labials and labialization are not mutually exclusive. (The features anterior and coronal also differentiate among other segments as well.)

The foregoing raises the question of formal notation and how primary and secondary articulation features should be differentiated from each other in a given segment. Chomsky and Halle did not formalize the relationship between primary and secondary articulation in terms of notation. An example would be the notation used for the labialized velar in contrast to the velarized labial. One of the questions in this context would be how many features relating to primary articulation could be replaced or had to be replaced by features relating to secondary articulation. In the example of the velarized labials, two features were replaced by their opposite value to indicate secondary articulation, and the low feature was dropped. In the case of the labialized velar, one feature was added (rounding), one feature was dropped (−low), two were retained (+high, +back), while one took its opposite value (−anterior).

Jakobson distinguished between pharyngeals and pharyngealization as follows. In the case of pharyngealization, the feature covering this phenomenon co-existed with other features. In contrast a single one was used to describe the phenomenon pharyngeality in the case of a pharyngeal (cf. above, p. 125). Chomsky and Halle in their classification (1968, p. 307) used a combination of three features to specify secondary articulation. As expected, the three features coincide with the respective three features of primary articulation. Based on the generalization that these secondary features (consisting of pharyngealization, palatalization, and velarization) did not co-occur with consonants formed with the body of the tongue (that is, with consonants which were specified as nonanterior and noncoronal), secondary articulation was specified by replacing the three final features used for primary articulation by the three features used for secondary articulation. Unfortunately, the above generalization, though neat, proved incorrect, and it is difficult to accommodate some facts about sounds found in natural languages within the resultant framework. The question arises, for example, how palatalized velars, pharyngealized velars, or pharyngealized palatals (which do seem to exist by their own account (cf. Chomsky and Halle, 1968, p. 170)) are to be handled.

Based on their own chart (1968, p. 307), Chomsky and Halle provided characterizations for certain sounds, as shown in Figure 8. In II and III, the palatal and the palatalized velar, and the pharyngeal and the pharyngealized velar, respectively, cannot be differentiated. The same would also hold true, of course, for pharyngealized palatals. It would seem clear that the Chomsky-Halle feature framework is not equipped to handle some of the distinctions represented by the sounds found in various languages.[81]

To remedy this situation a modification of the feature system would be required. Alternatively, a formal distinction between primary and secondary articulatory features would be needed.

	Anterior	Coronal	High	Low	Back
Given (I)					
Velar	−	−	+	−	+
Dental	+	+	−	−	−
Velarized dental	+	+	+	−	+
Given (II)					
Velar	−	−	+	−	+
Palatal	−	−	+	−	−
Palatalized velar (not given)	−	−	+	−	−
Given (III)					
Velar	−	−	+	−	+
Pharyngeal	−	−	−	+	+
Pharyngealized velar (not given)	−	−	−	+	+

Figure 8. Chomsky-Halle relationship between primary and secondary articulation.

The second alternative seems preferable, especially since secondary articulation does not replace primary articulation. Rather the features involved in primary articulation are also involved in secondary articulation, although quite frequently with opposite values.

A further point in the present framework pertains to the phonetic interpretation of the morphophonemic segments containing a secondary articulation parameter. Chomsky and Halle (1968, p. 223) posited the morphophonemes /k^w/, /g^w/, and /x^w/ for English. With respect to the interpretation of these segments as phonetic sequences, they stated:

> Among the velars, the stops are subdivided into [± round]; the labialized consonants are interpreted as the sequences [k^w], [g^w], and [x^w] respectively. The velar continuant /x/ becomes phonetic [h].[82]

Chomsky and Halle accomplished this interpretation as per the following rule:

$$\emptyset \rightarrow w \; \Big/ \begin{bmatrix} +\text{round} \\ C \end{bmatrix} \underline{\hspace{3cm}}$$

Realistically, rounding is extended from the previous segment to the segment at hand. However, the above rule does not adequately express this relationship. The rule should express the phonetic transformation of secondary articulation in one segment to primary articulation in the following phonetic segment. It seems clear that the phonetic interpretation given to rounding should also apply to other types of secondary articulations.

Obstruction Properties for Consonants

The properties or features considered uniquely vocalic (aperture) in the Trubetzkoyan framework have been already discussed. In the context of the three major coordinates to vowel and consonant quality outlined in *Grundzüge*, Trubetzkoy termed the properties or features that were specifically consonantal "properties based on the manner of overcoming an obstruction." He distinguished three types: properties based on the manner of overcoming an obstruction of the first degree, of the second degree, and of the third degree.[83] Below, this conceptualization is discussed.

Properties Based on the Manner of Overcoming an Obstruction of the First Degree   According to Trubetzkoy, the specific feature which separates the consonants from the vowels is the formation of an obstruction in the oral cavity and overcoming it.

He noted that the traditional classification in which consonants were categorized as occlusives, fricatives, and sonorants could be viewed in terms of degree of obstruction involved. The occlusives could be regarded as having the highest degree, the fricatives a medial degree, and the sonorants the lowest degree of obstruction without ever reaching the point where there was no obstruction. It will be recalled that for the vowels no obstruction was characteristic.[84]

Trubetzkoy contrasted the occlusives as *Momentanlaute* ("momentary sounds or stops") to the fricatives and sonorants as continuants, and the occlusives and fricatives as obstruents to the sonorants. The following demonstrates these relationships:

	Occlusives	Fricatives	Sonorants
$\pm$ Continuant	−	+	+
$\pm$ Obstruent	+	+	−

These sounds thus yielded five binary oppositions as follows:

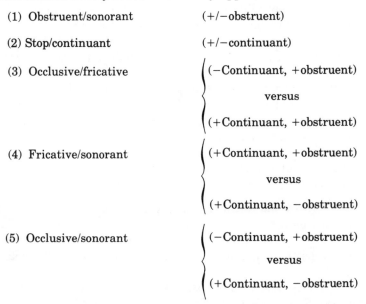

(1) Obstruent/sonorant   (+/−obstruent)

(2) Stop/continuant   (+/−continuant)

(3) Occlusive/fricative   (−Continuant, +obstruent)
                                    versus
                            (+Continuant, +obstruent)

(4) Fricative/sonorant   (+Continuant, +obstruent)
                                    versus
                            (+Continuant, −obstruent)

(5) Occlusive/sonorant   (−Continuant, +obstruent)
                                    versus
                            (+Continuant, −obstruent)

Not all three degrees of obstruction were always distinctive in a language. Trubetzkoy set up the following correlations, based on whether the three degrees of obstruction were distinctive in a particular language. These correlations were the:

1. *Correlation of sonants*[85]—Characterized the opposition between sonorants and obstruents. According to Trubetzkoy, the
   correlation of sonants is only present in those cases where the
   opposition between fricatives and occlusives is nonphonologi-
   cal in a given language. An example would be Tamil, which
   has five obstruents, variously realized depending on their
   context, and five sonorants: (/P, T, Ṭ, Č, K/ and /w, 1, ḷ, y, ɹ /
   (1939/1969, p. 142).
2. *Correlation of stops or continuants*—Presupposed that the opposition between fricatives and sonorants was nondistinctive
   in a language. Trubetzkoy observed that the first and second
   correlations did not occur very frequently. The correlation of
   stops or continuants in particular was hardly ever found in
   its pure form. It was usually the case that all three degrees of
   obstruction were distinctive in a language. When all three
   degrees of obstruction were distinctive, he spoke of the following three correlations:
3. *Correlation of constriction or occlusiveness*—Related to the
   distinctive opposition between occlusives and spirants. For
   example, the German contrasts /k-x/, /p̌-f/, and /č-š/ involve
   the opposition of constriction or occlusiveness. According to
   Trubetzkoy this opposition ranked among the most common
   correlations in the languages of the world.
4. *Correlation between fricatives and sonorants*—Illustrated by
   the opposition of /r/ and /ř/ in Czech, or the opposition between
   labial sonorants and voiced labial spirants found in Chichewa, a Bantu language.
5. *Correlation between occlusives and sonorants*—Found in languages that do not have spirants, for example, in Serbo-
   Croatian (Štokavian): /b:v/ = /d:1/ = /ḍ:ḷ/.

Trubetzkoy maintained that the distinction between occlusives and sonorants involved "Maximally different types of articulation . . . from an acoustic point of view." He therefore termed
this last type of opposition "correlation of contrast" (1939/1969, p.
144).

***Properties Based on the Manner of Overcoming an Obstruc-
tion of the Second Degree***   The above five distinctions were established by means of the two features +/− continuant, and +/−
obstruent. In addition Trubetzkoy also set up what he called *oppositions based on the manner of overcoming an obstruction of the
second degree*. These oppositions, which were also binary, related
to phonemes within the same degree of obstruction and which

also belonged to the same series of localization. These were the correlations of:

Tension
Intensity
Aspiration
Recursion
Release
Preaspiration
Voice

The question of redundancy arose in those cases where several of these secondary features co-occurred in the same segment. Language-internal criteria, such as the physical correlates of the archiphoneme, then determined which of these features actually was to be considered redundant. For example, if voicing and tensing occur in the same segment such that a voiced lenis is contrasted with a voiceless fortis, and a voiceless fortis appears in the position of neutralization, the voicing feature was considered distinctive. The determination of which feature was redundant depended on the minus value which appeared in the position of neutralization. Thus:

Fortis $\left\{ \begin{array}{l} (+\text{Tense}) \\ (-\text{Voice}) \end{array} \right.$ Lenis $\left\{ \begin{array}{l} (-\text{Tense}) \\ (+\text{Voice}) \end{array} \right.$
Voiceless   Voiced

Archiphoneme: $\left\{ \begin{array}{l} (+\text{Tense}) \\ (-\text{Voice}) \end{array} \right.$

However, if the plus and minus values of two features coincide and each could be potentially redundant, it was not clear which actually was to be considered redundant. The following example from Danish illustrates the point. In Danish aspirated fortis obstruents are opposed to unaspirated lenis obstruents. The unaspirated lenis occurs in the position of neutralization (thus: −aspirated, −tense).

The above approach is somewhat different from the position which Trubetzkoy had taken on the co-occurrence of features in vowels, when he had spoken of fused units (see p. 101 ff.). Contrary to Jakobson, neither feature could be considered redundant (for example, frontness and unroundedness, backness and roundedness; cf. above, p. 101 ff.).

Regarding properties based on the manner of overcoming an obstruction of the first degree and of the second degree,

Trubetzkoy considered the feature relating to the first degree as primary (that is, $+/-$ obstruent, $+/-$ continuant).

He also noted the following general tendencies with respect to the relationship between these two sets of features (of the first and second degree).

The first tendency is that the higher (greater) the degree of obstruction found in a consonant, the greater the differentiation by means of secondary features. The occlusives were thus more highly differentiated by secondary features than the fricatives, and the fricatives in turn were more highly differentiated than the sonorants. But this was only a general tendency. It was thus possible that the occlusives had two classes of sounds that were differentiated by such secondary features and that the fricatives and sonorants only had one such class. This is illustrated by Danish, where the occlusives have a voiced and voiceless class and the fricatives and sonorants have only one class /b-p, d-t, g-k, f-s/ and /r, l, v, δ, γ, m, n, ŋ/.

Trubetzkoy noted, however, that the languages in which occlusives and fricatives were divided into the same two classes and differentiated by the same secondary feature, were still the most common. German and English are examples in which the secondary feature of voicing divides both classes.

A second general tendency was the following. In cases where all three degrees of obstruction (occlusives, fricatives, and sonorants) were each divided into two classes, a different secondary feature generally divided each of the three degrees of obstruction. An illustration is Scottish-Gaelic (1939/1969, p. 149), where the occlusives are differentiated by aspiration, the fricatives by voice, and the sonorants by intensity. An exception to this tendency is Irish, in which voice differentiates among all three degrees of obstruction.

A third general tendency related to the correlation of constriction. In cases where a language has the correlation of constriction, that is, the opposition between occlusives and fricatives is distinctive and where the secondary voice feature is also distinctive for the occlusives and the fricatives, a three-member phoneme bundle is often found instead of the expected four phonemes. Trubetzkoy illustrated this with an example from Serbo-Croatian (Čakavian) which has /p-b/, /t-d/, /ţ-ḑ/, /v-f/, but /k-x-γ/, /c-s-z/, /č-š-ž/.

A fourth tendency related to occlusives. In instances where two secondary features are differentiated among the occlusives, one is either the aspiration feature or the recursion feature (ejective), the other is the tension feature or a fusion of the tension and the voice features.

Trubetzkoy also noted a close relationship between the recursion and the aspiration feature. He found that the "weak" member of the recursive opposition is generally aspirated (while the "strong" member is produced with a closed glottis). Conversely, with respect to the aspiration feature, the "strong" member was the one that was aspirated (1939/1969, p. 152). Trubetzkoy also observed that the presence of more than two secondary features in one phoneme is rare, for example, the East Caucasian languages, where a combination of the tension and voice features and the intensity and recursion feature is found. Avar thus had the following contrasts: /g-k-K-k'-K'/.

A fifth observation related to a general rule rather than a tendency, is that aspiration and constriction are, as Trubetzkoy observed, mutually exclusive.

A comparison of the above Trubetzkoyan classification with the Jakobsonian feature classification found in *Preliminaries* and *Fundamentals* discloses several interesting facts. The most important and consequential change found in the Jakobsonian classification has already been noted: Where the Trubetzkoyan classification differentiated properties which are specifically vocalic and those which are specifically consonantal, in the Jakobsonian classification the same features applied to consonants and vowels. (This is true at least of the general format of this theory, even though some features by their very nature remained specifically consonantal.)

In *Grundzüge* the first feature division is two-way, $+/-$ obstruction, grouping the phonemic system into consonants and vowels. The first division in the Jakobsonian classification is four-way, using two features which need to be considered together: consonantal/nonconsonantal and vocalic/nonvocalic. The phonological system is thereby classed into:

1. Liquids   (+vocalic, +consonantal)

2. Glides   (−vocalic, −consonantal)
   (including h)

3. Vowels   (+vocalic, −consonantal)

4. Consonants   (−vocalic, +consonantal)

In contrast with the above classication, Trubetzkoy had grouped the liquids and glides with the consonants and opposed them to the vowels.

The second distinction is that based on degrees of obstruction the classification in *Grundzüge* involved the two features +/− obstruent and +/− continuant. These two features yielded five possible oppositions for Trubetzkoy. Depending on the distinctive occurrence of a given opposition in a language, he established five different correlations (see above). Such a distinction in conception as well as terminology was not made by Jakobson. Once a feature is established, no further nomenclature was added to characterize specific feature co-occurrences.

Trubetzkoy distinguished between three degrees of obstruction related to the occlusives, fricatives, and the sonorants, differentiated by the features +/− obstruent and +/− continuant. In the Jakobsonian framework the feature +/− continuant (interrupted) is used as well. However, its application in the context of a segment is somewhat different. In *Grundzüge* the feature +/− continuant differentiated the occlusives from the fricatives and the sonorants. The liquids were considered part of the sonorants. For Jakobson, the liquids were established as a separate class by the consonantal/nonconsonantal and vocalic/nonvocalic dichotomies. Because of the primary ranking of the consonantal and vocalic features, +/− continuant in the Jakobsonian classification cuts across the liquids as well, and distinguishes /l/ as a continuant from /r/ as a noncontinuant. In the Trubetzkoyan framework, in which the continuant feature separated the occlusives from the fricatives and the sonorants, /r/ and /l/ were not differentiated by the feature +/−continuant. Both /r/ and /l/ belonged to the sonorant class.[86] Jakobson did not use the notion or term "sonorant" in his classification at all. An interesting comparison of the concept of sonorant as it is used in *Grundzüge* and *Sound Pattern* is presented later (p. 152 ff.).

A third difference between the Trubetzkoy and Jakobsonian classifications is that Trubetzkoy listed seven features based on the manner of overcoming an obstruction of the second degree (see above). Only the voice and the tensing features are listed in *Preliminaries* (p. 85).[87] The articulatory correlates of the tensing feature were described as follows:

> . . . tense vowels are articulated with a greater distinctness and pressure than the corresponding lax vowels. The muscular strain

affects the tongue, the wall of the vocal tract and the glottis. The higher tension is associated with greater deformation of the entire vocal tract from its neutral position. This is in agreement with the fact that tense phonemes have a longer duration than their lax counterparts. (Jakobson, Fant, and Halle, 1952, p. 38)

Jakobson, Fant and Halle further noted uncertainty about the acoustic effects related to the greater and lesser rigidity of the walls of the vocal tract and the glottis.

The opposition of release listed under the above category by Trubetzkoy may partially correspond to the checked/unchecked feature in the Jakobsonian framework. It will be recalled that Trubetzkoy had used the term "checked/unchecked" in conjunction with the vowels (see above p. 107, and note 60).

The remaining secondary features listed in *Grundzüge* do not appear in *Preliminaries* or *Fundamentals*. However, the following statement from *Fundamentals* may be examined in this context:

> The supposed multiplicity of features proves to be largely illusory. If two or more allegedly different features never co-occur in a language, and if they, furthermore, yield a common property, distinguishing them from all other features, then they are to be interpreted as different implementations of one and the same feature, each occurring to the exclusion of the other and, consequently presenting a particular case of complementary distribution. (Jakobson and Halle, 1956, p. 27)

Although Trubetzkoy considered the problem of redundancy in feature representation, he did not formulate a conception of feature economy or the associated notion of complementary distribution. Following the above guiding principle, Jakobson, by his own statement (Jakobson and Halle, 1956, p. 28), lumped into the tension feature four of the Trubetzkoyan secondary features, namely, the tension feature, the preaspiration feature, the aspiration feature, and the intensity or pressure feature.

This leaves the Trubetzkoyan recursion feature, which does not occur in the Jakobsonian framework. It is subsequently found in the Chomsky-Halle system (1968, p. 323) as a supplementary movement feature described under pressure or ejection.

Some additional remarks on the tension or tenseness feature are in order here. Trubetzkoy's tenseness feature (1931a) was included for both the consonants and the vowels. Its distinctiveness with respect to the vowels has been very much subject to reservation (see above, p. 73, and note 45). Also, its autonomous status in the Jakobsonian classification never seems to have been quite beyond doubt, although it at times stands strongly defended (cf. Jakobson and Halle, 1961). The opposition of tenseness also appeared in Jakobson and Lotz, *Notes on the French Phonemic Pattern* (1951/1962, p. 429), where it was defined as follows:

> . . . tense/lax, the former are produced with walls stiffened by muscular tension and the latter by lax articulation. The stiffening of the walls of the resonance chambers causes a more definite formant ("clangs" the sound), whereas a lax wall produces a great damping. (1949c/1962, p. 429)

And:

> The tense consonants (v. lax) demand not only stiffened walls but also a stronger airstream. (1949c/1962, p. 430)

The concepts of tenseness and laxness have had a long linguistic standing, though the differences between the two have been ascribed to various parts of the speech organs. Bell (1967) ascribed it to "differences in the behavior of the pharynx," Sweet (1906) approached it in terms of "shape of tongue," Heffner (1950) to "laryngeal positions and air pressures," and Sievers (1901) pointed out the parallelism of voicelessness and tension. (For further detail, see Jakobson and Halle, 1961.)

It is clear that the difficulty with tenseness and laxness does not involve its phonetic existence but rather its distinctive status. The problem of co-occurrence of two or more features with the opposition tense/lax, the resultant problem of the separability of these features, and the question of redundancy already discussed for the timbre features (see above, p. 102) are all magnified. Critical voices on the possibly general nature of its redundant character have never been completely stilled.

The frequent pairing of the tenseness feature with another feature, for example, voicelessness had been pointed out by Trubetzkoy for the stop consonants (1936c, pp. 14–15; also 1939/ 1969, p. 147 ff.). In connection with the oppositions voiced/ voiceless and fortis/lenis, Trubetzkoy observed that only one of these features needed to be abstracted as distinctive. Ivić (1965b, p. 76) similarly called attention to the frequent parallelism between the tenseness/laxness feature and the degree of vocalic aperture (cf. also Jakobson, Fant, and Halle, 1952, p. 36), duration, and aspiration. Ivić noted that the tenseness/laxness feature was "perhaps the most variegated as to its realizations in various languages and various types of sounds." He pointed out that there was no invariant mark of tenseness in the spectrum.

As to acoustic correlates, Jakobson and Halle (1963, p. 57) with respect to vowels had stated that a "tense vowel always displays a greater deviation from the neutral formant pattern." In *Fundamentals* tense/lax had been acoustically defined in terms of a "higher (v. lower) total amount of energy in conjunction with a greater (v. smaller) spread of the energy in the spectrum and in time" (p. 30).

The very nonspecific correlates given in Jakobson and Halle's *Tenseness and Laxness* (1961) were adopted by Chomsky and Halle in *Sound Pattern.* Chomsky and Halle specified the tenseness feature in terms of the manner in which "the entire articulatory gesture of a given sound is executed by the supraglottal musculature. . . ." Tense vowels here are "executed with a greater deviation from the neutral or rest position of the vocal tract . . ." (1968, p. 324).

For Trubetzkoy, tension had only included the opposition fortis/lenis. But in addition to the tension feature, he also posited an intensity (pressure) feature, an aspiration feature, and a preaspiration feature. As noted earlier, Jakobson collapsed all four of these features into the tension feature (1956, p. 38). Based on *Grundzüge,* the common denominator for these features can be sought in varying degrees and proportions of an increase in air pressure and buccal tensing (1939/1969, p. 145 ff.).

In an attempt to support the autonomous status of the tense/lax opposition, Jakobson, Fant, and Halle (1952, p. 38 ff.) pointed out that in some languages the features of voice and laxness do not coincide. Their examples included Suto, an African language, where aspiration only relates to unvoiced stops, and some Indian languages where aspiration only relates to voiced stops.

The opposition of aspiration had been subsumed in the opposition tense/lax in *Preliminaries.* As shown below, Chomsky and Halle in *Sound Pattern* again accorded it almost autonomous status. Their features were meant to represent the independently controllable movements of the vocal apparatus. They thus distinguished between tenseness in the supraglottal muscles (tenseness proper) and tenseness in the subglottal cavities (aspiration) since these are "controlled by a different mechanism." They labeled the feature relating to tension in the subglottal cavities as a feature of "heightened subglottal pressure." In addition to this feature, aspiration also required that "there be no constriction at the glottis" (1968, p. 326). (See below for a discussion of the features subsumed under the tenseness feature by Jakobson, as related to the Chomsky and Halle classification.)

Coming back to the comparison between Trubetzkoy and Jakobson the fourth Trubetzkoyan distinction, based on degree of obstruction, was that between fricatives and sonorants (or occlusives and sonorants). This distinction was formally absent from the Jakobsonian classification. Sonorants for Trubetzkoy included the liquids, glides, and nasals and had already been partly divided up by the consonantal and vocalic features in the Jakobsonian classification. This left the nasals, to which Jakobson contrasted the orals by a feature of nasality. It is of interest to note that Jakobson did not use the concept or term "sonorant" in any sense whatever in *Preliminaries* or *Fundamentals*.

The fifth distinction is that the nasals in the Trubetzkoyan classification were distinguished from the orals in terms of resonance, which constituted Trubetzkoy's third coordinate to consonant and vowel quality. Trubetzkoy characterized the nasals in terms of oral closure with a lowered velum. Unlike Jakobson, Trubetzkoy distinguished three different degrees of nasality:

1. *The opposition between nasals with complete oral closure and nasals with incomplete oral closure*—According to Trubetzkoy, this distinction functioned only rarely phonologically. Old Irish is said to have a contrast between nasals with complete and incomplete oral closure.

2. *The opposition between nasals with complete oral closure and orals (occlusives)*—Trubetzkoy termed this opposition "universal" and observed that, generally speaking, all localization series could have their own nasal. The laryngeal series constitutes an exception to this generalization. A further tendency with respect to the nasals concerned the correlation of constriction (that is, the opposition between occlusives and fricatives). Trubetzkoy noted that fricatives and nasals were frequently mutually exclusive in the same localization series. An illustration from Avar exemplifies what is meant: /p-m/, and /t-n/, but /k-x/, /ḳ-x̱/, /č-š/, /ɣ-1/. Trubetzkoy called the opposition between nasals and orals the *correlation of nasals*. For the vowels, the opposition between nasalized and

non-nasalized vowels was termed the *correlation of nasaliza-tion*. Even though nasals involve oral closure, nasals in the Trubetzkoyan classification were always sonorants, that is, "consonants with a minimal degree of obstruction, for the egress of air through the nose, which is made possible by lowering the velum, renders the oral closure ineffective" (1939/1969, p. 168 ff.).

3. *The correlation of seminasals or the correlation of consonantal nasalization*—This correlation is posited for languages in which, in addition to the opposition nasal/oral, a second op-position between "nasalized implosion and non-nasalized plo-sive release" exists:

> Such semi-nasalized occlusives give the impression acoustically of being combinations of a very short nasal and an occlusive. They can exist as separate phonemes only, if in the given language they are phonologically distinguished from normal (non-nasalized) occlu-sives on the one hand, and from combinations of "nasal plus occlu-sive" on the other. (Trubetzkoy, 1939/1969, p. 169)

Ful, an African language, constituted an example. It has /b, d, g, ɟ/, and semi-nasalized /ɓ, ɗ, g̃/, and ɟ̃/ as independent phonemes, in addition to the nasals /n, m, ŋ, and ɲ/, and the nasal combina-tions /mb, nd, ŋg/ and ɲɟ/.

In conjunction with these sounds, Trubetzkoy made the fol-lowing distinctions:

> While the true nasals are sonorants and consequently continuants, the "semi-nasals" may be considered stops. The relationship b:m etc. may be equated with the relation stop:continuant. In a language in which this relation is found, m, n, ŋ and ɲ must be termed "nasal continuants" and (ɓ, ɗ, g̃, and ɟ̃/ "nasal stops."[88] (1939/1969, p. 169)

Chomsky and Halle (1968) also were aware of the existence of this third distinction, in addition to the opposition nasal/non-nasal. They spoke of prenasalized consonants. However, the over-all distinctions made in the Chomsky-Halle classification are somewhat different. Like Trubetzkoy, Chomsky and Halle op-posed the nasals to the non-nasals as sounds "produced with a lowered velum which allows the air to escape through the nose" to sounds "produced with a raised velum so that the air from the lungs can escape only through the mouth" (1968, p. 316). How-ever, they considered nasalization as "superimposed upon a plosive articulation." In contrast, the nasals belonged to the sonorants in the Trubetzkoyan classification. The sonorants and the plosives were mutually exclusive, distinguished from each other as follows by degree of obstruction:

Plosive	Sonorant
+Obstruent	−Obstruent
−Continuant	+Continuant

Hence, the very framework of the Trubetzkoyan classification disallowed the consideration of the nasals as occlusives with a superimposed feature of nasalization. However, the same division of consonants into +/− obstruent also made it possible for Trubetzkoy to consider the "prenasalized consonants" as "nasalized plosives."

Chomsky and Halle, after Ladefoged (1964), noted that nasalization could also be found with affricates. Their example, taken from Ladefoged,[89] comes from Tiv (a West African language). They further noted that examples of simultaneous nasalization with continuants such as /z/ and /v/ were not known to them.

Trubetzkoy did not mention the co-occurrence of nasalization with affricates. However, he did cite an example of nasalization co-occurring with fricatives (1939/1969, p. 169). In conformity with the above division (+/−obstruent), these nasalized fricatives were included in the correlation of seminasals. Trubetzkoy cited as an example Chichewa (a North American Indian language), where, in addition to the seminasal stops /b̰, d̰, g̰, ɜ̰, ȝ̰/ the seminasal fricatives /ṽ, f̰/ and z̰, s̰/ exist.

By considering nasalization as superimposed "upon a plosive articulation," Chomsky and Halle could not handle prenasalized consonants as nasalized stops. They made the following distinction between prenasalized and nasal consonants:

> Phonetically, prenasalized consonants differ from the more familiar type of nasal consonants in that *the velum, which is lowered during the period of oral occlusion, is raised prior to the release of the oral occlusion,* whereas in the more common type of nasal consonant, the velum is raised simultaneously with or after the release of the oral occlusion. (1968, p. 317; emphasis added)

Chomsky and Halle suggested that it may be necessary to establish a feature "that governs timing of different movements within the limits of a single segment." As an alternative the possibility of considering the distinction between prenasalized and nasalized consonants as a distinction between delayed and instantaneous release was also noted.

Going back to the distinctions between Jakobson and Trubetzkoy, as just mentioned, the Jakobsonian classification did not contain a category of sounds labeled sonorants. Comparing the Chomsky-Halle classification to the classifications of Trubetzkoy and Jakobson shows that Chomsky and Halle posited what they called three major class features: vocalic, consonantal, and sonorant. Each of these major class features focused "on a different aspect of the open v. closed phase" of articulation (Chomsky and Halle, 1968, p. 302). The Chomsky-Halle major class features divided speech sounds into vowels, consonants, obstruents, sonorants, glides, and liquids.

It seems clear that the Chomsky-Halle classification shares several common characteristics with the classification given by Trubetzkoy. First, as did Trubetzkoy, Chomsky and Halle also operated with the opposition sonorant/obstruent. Sonorants were defined as "sounds produced with a vocal tract cavity configuration in which spontaneous voicing is possible," and obstruents are produced "with a cavity configuration that makes spontaneous voicing impossible" (1968, p. 302). Voicing here was related to constriction: "sounds formed with a more radical constriction than glides are nonsonorants." In accordance with the above definition, stops, fricatives, and affricates then are nonsonorants, while vowels, glides, nasal consonants, and liquids are sonorants. In the Trubetzkoyan classification vowels were not considered sonorants. Figure 9 illustrates the differences in the two classifications.

In conformity with Jakobson, but in contrast to Trubetzkoy, the glides for Chomsky and Halle also included /ʔ/ and /h/. They were thus also considered sonorants, while in the Trubetzkoyan classification they had been considered obstruents.[90]

In the Chomsky-Halle classification the oppositions vocalic/nonvocalic and consonantal/nonconsonantal only applied after the primary sonorant/nonsonorant division. Figure 10 shows how Chomsky and Halle distinguished among the sonorants.

The Chomsky-Halle classification also included a voiceless vowel which was differentiated from the voiced vowel by means of the opposition vocalic/nonvocalic. This distinction previously had

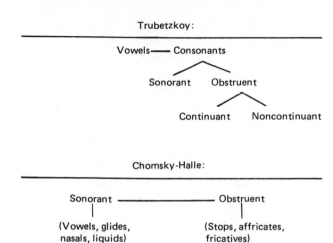

Figure 9. Differences between the Trubetzkoyan and the Chomsky-Halle classifications.

been used by Jakobson to separate the glides, which Jakobson had characterized as −consonantal, −vocalic. Chomsky and Halle retained the feature nonvocalic for the glides as well (1968, p. 303), so that voiceless vowels and glides could not be differentiated by the above three features (sonorant, vocalic, consonantal).

In summary, the differences in the use of the opposition +/− obstruent (= +/− sonorant) between Trubetzkoy and Chomsky-Halle can be stated as follows. In the Trubetzkoyan classification the major division existed between consonants and vowels. The

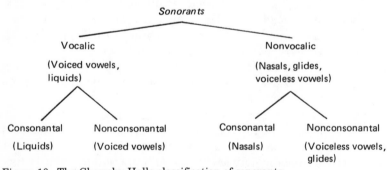

Figure 10. The Chomsky-Halle classification of sonorants.

dichotomies +/− obstruent and +/− continuant only applied to the subclassification of the consonants. Consequently, voiced and voiceless vowels could not be included as sonorants. The same was true for the glides /h/ and /ʔ/ (in the Jakobsonian and Chomsky-Halle conception). /h/ and /ʔ/ were considered obstruents by Trubetzkoy.

For Chomsky and Halle each of the three major class features, sonorant, vocalic, and consonantal, focused on a different aspect of the open versus closed phase. In the Trubetzkoyan classification the open versus close parameter related only to the consonant/vowel dichotomy. For the obstruent/sonorant classification and the continuant/noncontinuant classification, on the other hand, degree of obstruction was essential. It seems obvious, however that the articulatory criteria pertaining to the degree of obstruction and "the open v. close phase" parameters can be considered related.

The above conception reveals that the use of the term "sonorant" is not the same as its traditional use in the literature. *Sonante* ("sonorant") is defined by Marouzeau (1933) as follows:

> More specifically, this label is reserved for phonemes which simultaneously possess the oral resonance characteristics of vowels and the expiratory noise characteristics of consonants. The opposition of sonorant and consonant does not correspond to that between vowels and consonants. *The two latter terms designate the type, the former two the function.* . . . In a general sense, but especially in Indo-European grammar, [a sonorant is] *any consonant which can serve as a syllable nucleus,* that is, which can serve as a support for other consonants . . . (p. 209; emphasis added)

Chomsky and Halle (1968, p. 353 ff.) proposed to replace the major class features sonorant, vocalic, and consonantal by the features sonorant, syllabic, and consonantal since certain symmetrical relationships between specific rules could not be expressed by the former features. By replacing the feature vocalic by the feature syllabic, the segments constituting a syllabic peak could then be characterized. A division into the features sonorant, syllabic, and consonantal would set apart the obstruents as never performing syllabic function, but being syllabic under special circumstances. The classificatory changes shown in Table 16 would thus take place.

The following observations are in order with respect to the second classification in Table 16: 1) in order to operate with the notion syllabic peak, the notion of syllable ought to be defined;

Table 16.   Chomsky-Halle classificatory changes

	Feature		
	Sonorant	Consonantal	Vocalic
(I) *Sound Pattern* (p. 303)			
Voiced vowels	+	−	+
Voiceless vowels	+	−	−
Glides (I) /w, y/	+	−	−
Glides (II) /h, ʔ /	+	−	−
Liquids	+	+	+
Nasal consonants	+	+	−
Non-nasal consonants	−	+	−
	Sonorant	Syllabic	Consonantal
(II) *Sound Pattern* (p. 354)			
Vowels	+	+	−
Syllabic liquids	+	+	+
Syllabic glides	+	+	+
Syllabic nasals	+	+	+
Nonsyllabic liquids	+	−	+
Nonsyllabic nasals	+	−	+
Glides /w, y, h, ʔ /	+	−	−
Obstruents	−	−	+

and 2) the major class features in part I were defined in articulatory terms of aperture/closure. This is not the case for the features listed under II. The criteria utilized here relate to function as syllable peak (for the features sonorant, syllabic, and obstruent, but not for the feature consonantal). It may be argued that since the phonetic features are to represent the "phonetic capabilities of man" as Chomsky and Halle claim, and the rest of the features are classified in articulatory terms, articulatory criteria should be used consistently for the division into major class features. Instead a functional parameter is brought into play.

Like Trubetzkoy, Chomsky and Halle considered the feature +/− continuant as a subclass of the manner of articulation. They defined the feature +continuant articulatorily as follows: "the primary constriction in the vocal tract is not narrowed to the point where the airflow past the constriction is blocked." The feature −continuant is defined as "the airflow through the mouth is effectively blocked" (1968, p. 317 ff.).

The Chomsky-Halle classification of the liquids and glides is affected by this feature. It differs from that of Jakobson in that for the latter, [r] was considered interrupted, while [l] was continuant. As noted earlier, the Trubetzkoyan classification included [l] and [r] in the class of sonorants. [l] and [r] were thus considered continuants.

Chomsky and Halle called the earlier feature status of the liquids [r] and [l] into doubt. They distinguished a fricative [r], which they considered a continuant. As for the trilled [r], they considered the trill secondary. It "narrows the cavity without actually blocking the flow of air." They concluded that "consequently there was good reason to view trilled [r] as a continuant rather than a stop." As for the stop [r] they observed:

> ... the distinction between the tap [r] and the trilled [r] is produced by a difference in subglottal pressure: the trilled [r] is produced with heightened subglottal pressure, the tap [r] without it. (1968, p. 318)

Whether the [l] was to be considered a stop or continuant depended on their definition of a stop. If the correlate of a stop was total blockage of airflow, then [l] was a continuant and distinguished from [r] by a feature of laterality. (It is noteworthy that Trubetzkoy had used this to distinguish [l] and [r] (1939/1969, p. 139).) In contrast, if the articulatory correlate of a stop was the "blockage of airflow past primary stricture," the [l] had to be included in the stops. Chomsky and Halle suggested that classifying the [l] into the continuant/noncontinuant dichotomy should be based best on its behavior in a given language.

It is of interest to compare the Trubetzkoyan classification of properties based on the manner of overcoming an obstruction of the second degree with its equivalents in the Chomsky-Halle classification. Trubetzkoy had mentioned seven features under this rubric: the correlations of tension, intensity, aspiration, recursion, release, preaspiration, and voice (see above, p. 140).

Of these seven features, the Chomsky-Halle classification includes three: tension, voicing, and recursion (ejective). Trubetzkoy's aspiration feature is not listed by Chomsky and Halle. However, an equivalent feature can be found in heightened subglottal pressure, although Chomsky and Halle recognized that this feature in itself is not sufficient to account for aspiration. Aspiration also requires the absence of glottal constriction. In addition, preaspiration, mentioned by Trubetzkoy as a possible feature for some American Indian languages, for example, Fox and Hopi, was not listed by Chomsky and Halle. For Trubetzkoy, it opposed consonants with aspirate implosion to consonants without such implosion. He had not been quite certain whether feature status should be accorded to this phenomenon. The alternative was to consider the preaspirated consonants in these languages as a combination of two phonemes (/h/ + consonant). As noted earlier Jakobson considered this contrast an aspect of the tension feature (Jakobson and Halle, 1956, p. 29).

Chomsky and Halle did not mention preaspirated consonants either. It is conceivable that in their framework preaspirated consonants, like the aspirates, would be considered in terms of heightened subglottal pressure, absence of glottal constriction, and "a feature that governs the timing of different movements within the limits of a single segment." The possible existence of such a feature had been mentioned in conjunction with the prenasalized consonants.

Judging from the examples for Ful (1939/1969, p. 155), Trubetzkoy's release feature relates to the opposition between implosives and nonimplosives. In the Chomsky-Halle framework the implosives were characterized by glottal constriction and suction.

The last of Trubetzkoy's features, intensity (pressure), does not appear to have a direct equivalent in the Chomsky-Halle framework. This feature seems to resemble the Chomsky-Halle tenseness feature and possibly also their heightened subglottal pressure feature. Trubetzkoy defined the intensity or pressure feature with reference to the relation between resistance and air pressure:

> . . . when the muscles of the buccal organs are being relaxed, the air pressure is too strong. Hence the short duration and possible aspiration of the weak opposition members. When the buccal muscles are being tensed, the air pressure seems just about able to accomplish its task. Hence the relative length, the lack of aspiration, and the fact that the obstruction is overcome with great effort in the case of the strong opposition members. (Trubetzkoy, 1939/1969, p. 145)

CONCLUSION

The details of the Chomsky-Halle feature framework approximated those of the Trubetzkoyan classification more closely than did Jakobson's. The Jakobsonian features included neither implosives nor ejectives. It seems, however, that the feature checked/unchecked (physical correlate: with compression or closure of the glottis) appears to cut across the implosives and ejectives. Jakobson also reduced the features of tension, intensity, aspiration, and preaspiration to one feature, that of tension. It is important to repeat that Jakobson reduced these to one, based on interlanguage complementary distribution and a common denominator.

Jakobson's features were distinctive in the true sense of the word, the outgrowth of the functional orientation of the Prague School. After Jakobson came to the United States, the functionalism inherent in the distinctive feature concept was married to the criterion of economy. This may perhaps constitute a reflection of the influence of American distributionalism. Jakobson strove to reduce the number of his features according to these principles. He extended the criterion of complementary distribution from the constraints governing features within a language to constraints on features from a universal point of view. Trubetzkoy did not strive for economy based on such universal constraints. He did not make any concerted attempt to reduce the number of features. This accounts for the fact that, for example, he listed four features where Jakobson only listed one. Trubetzkoy stayed more closely to phonetic reality. Nevertheless, in both cases the features were distinctive in the Praguian sense.

In contrast, the Chomsky-Halle feature framework has shifted. The features established and listed in *Sound Pattern* are not specifically segregated based on their distinctive function. The goal of the Chomsky-Halle feature framework is approached from a somewhat different point of view: features in their framework are established with the aim of describing the "independently controllable aspects of the speech event." We read:

> There are therefore as many phonetic features as there are aspects under partially independent control. It is in this sense that the totality of phonetic features can be said to represent the speech-producing capabilities of the human vocal apparatus. (1968, p. 297)

The issue to be raised is how the "speech-producing capabilities of the human vocal apparatus" relate to the concept of distinctiveness. Are all those features, isolated based on this criterion, also distinctive? The answer must clearly be no. The following example illustrates the point. Chomsky and Halle established a suction feature, which in many languages is con-

comitant to click production, even though "apparently in no language are there contrasting pairs of utterances that differ solely
by this feature" (1968, p. 298). Chomsky and Halle accorded it
feature status because "click-like suction is clearly an independently controllable aspect of the speech event."

Trubetzkoy had also recognized the suction element as a
phonetic feature in connection with clicks. In contrast to
Chomsky and Halle, however, he did not accord it distinctive
status, and it does not appear as a feature in his classification. In
comparison with the earlier positions of Trubetzkoy and Jakobson, but in particular of Jakobson, features now hugged the
phonetic ground more closely.

The Chomsky and Halle features are also presumed to be
psychologically real. They claimed (1968, p. 294) that a phonetic
transcription is to be understood "not as a direct record of the
speech signal, but rather *as a representation of what the speaker of
a language takes to be the phonetic properties of a language*" (emphasis added), and ". . . the phonetic transcription, in this sense,
represents the speaker-hearer's interpretation rather than directly observable properties of the signal. . . ."

There are now three criteria with respect to features: their
distinctiveness, that they represent independently controllable
aspects of the vocal apparatus, and their psychological reality. It
would seem that psychological reality, in the above sense, has
always played a role in phonetic transcriptions, although it may
not have been made explicit in so many words. For example, in
the Praguian dichotomy between phonetics and phonology, an
interrelation had been considered natural between the base elements of the two disciplines. Although such a relationship had
not been stated explicitly in terms of psychological reality, it
could be interpreted in such terms. It would also appear that any
selection criteria operating in a gross phonetic transcription
would appear to have its roots in psychological reality.

The Chomsky-Halle features seem to relate to psychological
reality in two ways: in terms of the signal itself and in terms of
the physical correlates of the signal. Can it be said, for example,
that psychological reality is also commensurate with the independently controllable movements of the vocal apparatus? If
psychological reality were to apply to such movements, it would
seem very difficult to prove that the physical correlate of a feature
is felt as psychologically real as well. For example, is the physical

correlate of the feature heightened subglottal pressure or the feature anterior really psychologically real to a speaker (or hearer)?

Mentalistic terminology and definitions abounded in early Prague development in the context of the development of the distinctive feature concept, with ample reference to linguistic consciousness. However, the Praguians soon tried to rid their definitions of allusions to linguistic consciousness and related terminology. The reason can be sought in the fact that early Prague phonologists meant to establish linguistics as a scientific discipline. They were well aware that the concept of linguistic consciousness presented problems, that there was no method for studying it, nor was there any objective proof for the mentalistic claims in the earlier definitions.

In *Grundzüge* (1939/1969, p. 38), Trubetzkoy mentioned some of the reasons why this mentalistic approach relating to the phoneme concept was abandoned. There was no way to prove, for example, that all members of the speech community agreed upon or had the "same" linguistic consciousness. Furthermore, it was incorrect to attribute psychological reality to the phonemes only and not to speech sounds. Interpreted in terms of distinctiveness and nondistinctiveness of features, Trubetzkoy's statement could mean that all features have psychological reality, not only those that are distinctive. But since the Praguians were interested in isolating only the distinctive features, the concept of psychological reality was of no help. However, even though a definite effort was made by the Prague School to rid their phonological studies of mentalistic bias and allusions to linguistic consciousness, linguistic consciousness as an underlying force never seemed to have lost ground in Prague conceptual development. In Trubetzkoy's *Grundzüge*, for example, there is still sufficient mention of linguistic consciousness. The dilemma for Prague phonologists was that they could see no reasonable way to incorporate the concept into their theories. Thus the concept of distinctive features actually developed as a functional concept.

Chomsky and Halle essentially faced the same problem the Praguians did with respect to psychological reality. However, they did not consider the difficulty in objectively studying the concept as a reason to abandon it. Instead, they viewed psychological reality as a hypothetical base from which to proceed. There seems no doubt that an acceptable correspondence between their two criteria, psychological reality and independently controllable movements, will be fraught with problems. The extent to which such a correspondence can be established for individual features will also be certain to vary.

In addition to differences noted in their respective feature frameworks, a few overall thoughts should be recapitulated with respect to Trubetzkoy, Jakobson, and Chomsky and Halle. It is reasonable to claim that during the early development of feature theory, there was a preoccupation with abstracting and segregating distinctive features. Such an objective was closely related to typological studies and the discovery of universal laws about languages. Preoccupation with binarity had not yet become a major concern. Trubetzkoy and the early Jakobson are associated with this period of early development.

A second period was signaled by Jakobson's work in the United States and his collaboration with Fant and Halle. This was a period in which information theory and instrumental acoustics had a crucial impact on the direction of Jakobsonian thought. Binarity and economy of features became outstanding characteristics of this period. Most important, this period was also crowned by efforts to correlate features with instrumental acoustic findings. Both in the earlier and in this second period there was a concerted effort to express by means of distinctive features certain regularities and relationships found in a given language and certain generalizations which could be made about language in general. The emphasis and direction in which such generalizations were expressed varied.

We already discussed the general shift in the Chomsky-Halle feature framework. It appears that in the current model, too, major emphasis is given to establishing a feature framework best suited and capable of representing the highest number of regularities and generalizations found in a given language. Accordingly, in the Chomsky-Halle framework not three but four criteria had to be considered in the establishment of features: 1) their relation to distinctiveness, 2) their relation to psychological reality, 3) their relation to the independently controllable movements of the vocal apparatus, and 4) their capability to express the greatest number of generalizations most satisfactorily.

Although, ideally, it would be desirable to have a distinctive feature system capable of expressing all these aspects, ideal results seem difficult to obtain.

An additional point deserves discussion. This is the question regarding how, in the development of generative phonology, all the above requirements came to be associated with the distinctive feature concept. It is also of interest to trace this change in feature concept within generative phonology itself. As is known, Morris Halle was a student of Jakobson and he collaborated with his teacher on both *Preliminaries* and *Fundamentals*. He thus signaled agreement with the features as they appeared in these works. Halle also collaborated with Chomsky in *The Sound Pattern of English,* in which a major change in feature theory took place.

In the *The Sound Pattern of Russian* (1959), Halle connected the idea of distinctive features with the morphophoneme. He disassociated himself from taxonomic phonemics in favor of morphophonemics (or systematic phonemics). The morphophoneme, as discussed earlier (see above, p. 19 ff.), was seen by Halle as an extension of the Praguian notions of archiphoneme and morphophoneme and as connected with the Bloomfieldian basic (underlying) form. The disinterest in phonological discovery procedures which Halle demonstrated in his writing may in some way be connected with his awareness of the fact that distinctive features were originally most closely related to the phoneme concept. A disavowal of the relevance and importance of phonological discovery procedures at the level of the phoneme liberated the distinctive feature from the phoneme concept. The feature concept thus was set free to operate independently of the phoneme in the context of the morphophoneme. It is noteworthy that neither in *Preliminaries* nor in *Fundamentals* any reference was made to phonological discovery procedures. It almost seems that the phoneme had already lost its place in linguistic description in *Fundamentals* since in this work Jakobson only recognized a semantic level (morpheme to utterance) and a feature level (pp. 3−4). But the phoneme is accorded some status in the statement that:

> If the distinctive function of speech sounds is the only one under analysis, we use the so-called broad or phonemic transcription that denotes nothing but phonemes. (Jakobson and Halle, 1956, p. 10)

The feature framework of *The Sound Pattern of Russian* (1959) is Jakobsonian. Halle here operated strictly in binary terms, as laid out in his article, *In Defense of the Number Two* (1957). Even though Halle voiced reluctance to tamper with the Jakobsonian theoretical framework of distinctive features, in the *Sound Pattern of Russian* he changed the feature "plain" in the opposition flat/plain to "natural." He did so to avoid confusion with respect to the opposition sharp/plain. He also maintained that the oppositions consonantal/nonconsonantal and vocalic/ nonvocalic were linked more closely than were the other features. He considered these two oppositions to be different from the other features in that all morphophonemes had to have them. In other words, Halle argued that these two features were distinctive for all morphophonemes. In terms of the simplicity metric, they "are the only features that have no zeros." However, unlike the other features, they "do not generally function as distinctive marks" (1959, p. 52). Distinctive mark, in contrast to distinctive feature, was to be interpreted as the property that actually differentates two morphophonemes. Halle related the two oppositions to the notion of simplicity and generality of linguistic statements. These notions had been expressed in his condition (4) governing phonological statements:

> . . . the phonological description must be appropriately integrated into the grammar of the language. Particularly in selecting phonological representations of individual morphemes, these must be chosen so as to yield simple statements of all grammatical operations—like inflection and derivation—in which they may be involved. (Halle, 1959, p. 24)

Halle discussed the possibility of replacing the two features from the point of view of code efficiency and pointed out that they were part of the theoretical framework of phonology. He concluded that a change with respect to these two features would *"in effect be a proposal to modify the underlying theory itself—a step to be undertaken only for the most cogent reasons"* (Halle, 1959, p. 53; emphasis added).

Although Halle introduced the concept of the morphophoneme into generative phonology, *The Sound Pattern of Russian* clearly attests that at the time he wrote this work he still steadfastly operated within the Jakobsonian feature framework.

In *On the Bases of Phonology* (1964) Halle still adhered to the feature framework of *Preliminaries* and *Fundamentals* although acoustic feature correlates were omitted and the articulatory correlates experienced a number of changes as well. (In this context, also compare note 61 with respect to his use of different degrees of narrowing of the vocal tract, and the terms "contact," "occlusion," "obstruction," and "constriction.") The following statement found in *On the Bases of Phonology* deserves attention:

If it is true that a small set of attributes suffices to describe the phonetic properties of all languages of the world, then it would appear quite likely *that these attributes are connected with something fairly basic in man's constitution,* something which is quite independent of his cultural background. (Halle, 1964, p. 329; emphasis added)

Halle notes that the phonetic attributes might be of interest to psychologists because of their potential as productive parameters in the description of auditory stimuli in general. But for linguistics:

. . . the lack of psychological work in this area is not fatal. *For the linguist it suffices if the attributes selected yield reasonable, elegant, and insightful descriptions of all relevant linguistic data. And this in fact they accomplish.* (ibid.; emphasis added)

Halle appeared to address two issues in this statement. On the one hand he attempted to relate features to something "basic in man's constitution." (Taken by itself, this statement seems somewhat ambiguous, since it may refer to the physical (vocal apparatus) or to the mental aspect of speech production.) This aspect was also stressed by Chomsky. On the other hand, Halle reiterated the Jakobsonian principles related to feature theory. Jacobson probably would not have disagreed with the first part of Halle's statement. However, it would seem that Jakobson was not able to integrate the two characterizations within a single two-dimensional framework. He therefore chose to concentrate on the second part of Halle's statement regarding the criteria for feature selection, when he developed his distinctive features in *Preliminaries* and *Fundamentals*.

In *Kindersprache, Aphasie und allgemeine Lautgesetze* (1942/1962d), in the context of first language acquisition Jakobson claimed that the contrast consonant-vowel is the most basic in the acquisition process, although his feature dichotomies consonantal/nonconsonantal and vocalic/nonvocalic were not representative of this fact. Jakobson also accommodated the liquids and the glides in these two features and commented that the liquids were acquired relatively late in a child's language. From a simplicity and generality point of view the division into four groups, consonants, vowels, liquids, and glides, is to be preferred. Halle points to the merits of such a division in *The Sound Pattern of Russian.*

Another example is the opposition oral/nasal. Jakobson counted this opposition among the primary features acquired first by children, although only for the consonants. The oral/nasal contrast is acquired relatively late for the vowels. The Jakobsonian framework again was not expressive of this fact. The opposition between nasals and obstruents and that of nasalized vowels and non-nasalized vowels was expressed by one feature, oral/nasal. Jakobson associated nasality in vowels with a more complicated production and also pointed to the occurrence of nasalized vowels in general. These points were taken up in the subsequent theory of markedness.

In *On the Bases of Phonology,* Halle also called attention to the dual function of the distinctive features:

> On the one hand *they have been used to characterize different aspects of vocal tract behavior,* such as the location of the different narrowings in the vocal tract . . . . On the other hand, *the features have functioned as abstract markers for the designation of individual morphemes.* It is necessary at this point to give an account of how this dual function of the feature is built into the theory. (1964, p. 332; emphasis added)

As can be seen, the previous "articulatory correlate" of a feature had now evolved to being considered *as a second purpose of the feature,* namely, "to characterize different aspects of vocal tract behavior." Here then the relationship between the phonetic aspect of a feature and its abstract use are juxtaposed and becomes an issue and will remain one in subsequent feature development. This contrasts sharply with the earlier feature conception.

In Prague phonology, even though the (articulatory or acoustic) correlates of the features had been stated, the features themselves, when distinctive, had been considered phonological abstractions. However, features could be distinctive in one language and nondistinctive (or simply phonetic) in another. In generative phonology, phonetic representation became part of the model. The problem of what happens to the distinctive feature on the phonetic level therefore has to be dealt with. This was not the case for the Praguians.

Already in *On the Bases of Phonology,* Halle maintained that not all binary features need to be binary on the phonetic level. To quote:

... the phonological component will include rules replacing some of the pluses and minuses in the matrices by integers representing the different degrees of intensity which the feature manifests in the utterance. (1964, p. 333)

Halle considered that the assignment of a "phonetic interpretation to phonemic matrices is *uniform for all languages*" (p. 333; emphasis added) and reflects the fact that:

> ... *the articulatory apparatus of man is the same everywhere, that men everywhere are capable of controlling the same few aspects of their vocal tract behavior. The phonetic features represent therefore, the capacities of man to produce speech sounds and constitute, in this sense, the universal phonetic framework of language.* (1964, p. 333; emphasis added)

Here then, still within the Jakobsonian framework is what must be considered a programmatic statement with respect to the features of *The Sound Pattern of English.*

Taken together with a pronouncement from Chomsky's *Current Issues in Linguistic Theory,* the above may be taken to supply the rest of the prerequisites for the new direction in feature development:

> There is no reason why the linguist must necessarily limit himself to "the study of phenomena and their correlations," avoiding any attempt to gain insight into such data by means of an explanatory theory of language, a theory, which is, of course, "mentalistic" in that it deals with the character of mental activity rather than with its physical basis.[91] (1964, p. 106)

So far nothing has been said specifically about prosodic features. For Trubetzkoy they had formed a separate class in *Grundzüge.* Some discussion of them had been included in Jakobson's *Fundamentals* but not in his earlier *Preliminaries.* Prosodic features have always presented an extremely challenging topic. However, recent research in this area has not kept abreast with the interest and progress in the rest of the feature spectrum.

Chomsky and Halle omitted the prosodic features from *The Sound Pattern of English* with the observation that "the investigation of these features had not progressed to a point where a discussion in print would be useful" (p. 329). However, their omission should not be interpreted as an expression of an earlier neglect of prosodic features by the Prague School by either Trubetzkoy or Jakobson. On the contrary, the interest in prosodic phenomena is as old as the interest in other features. In fact, preoccupation with prosodic phenomena predated preoccupation with other distinctive features and actually gave impetus to the crystallization of these features.

To round out the feature picture, a cursory comparison of the prosodic oppositions of Trubetzkoy's *Grundzüge* and Jakobson's *Fundamentals* is presented in the appendices. The comparison is also representative of the status of the prosodic features at the end of the "golden era" of Prague phonology and of their further consolidation and systematization with the aid of acoustic instrumentation in the Jakobsonian framework.

APPENDICES

The Prosodic
Oppositions of
Grundzüge and
Fundamentals:
A Cursory Comparison

Trubetzkoy made three major distinctions regarding prosodic oppositions.

First, he recognized two types of prosodic units or prosodemes depending on whether or not a syllable nucleus could be divided into even smaller prosodic units. He defined the syllable nucleus as "that portion of a syllable which, in accordance with the laws of the particular language, carries the distinctive prosodic properties" (1939/1969, p. 170).

Syllable nuclei could consist of: (1) a vowel, (2) a vowel combination, (3) a consonant, or (4) a combination of vowel plus consonant.

The prosodic unit which was smaller than the syllable nucleus and formed a part of the syllable nucleus was called a "mora." Whether a language utilizes the syllable (nucleus in toto) or the mora as a prosodic unit depends on the structural laws of each language. Trubetzkoy divided languages into syllable-counting languages and mora-counting languages.

Second, Trubetzkoy made an additional distinction between culminative and nonculminative prosodic oppositions. Culminative oppositions had the following phonetic correlates: (1) an increase in expiratory force, (2) a rise in pitch, (3) lengthening, and (4) more emphatic articulation.

The phonetic correlates of culminative oppositions were distributed as follows, depending on whether they related to syllable-counting or mora-counting languages: (1) an increase in force in syllable-counting languages, (2) a rise in pitch in mora-counting languages, (3) lengthening in both syllable-counting and mora-counting languages. Trubetzkoy did not give specifics with respect to what he termed more emphatic articulation.

Third, Trubetzkoy further divided prosodic properties into: (1) differential prosodic properties *(Differenzierungseigenschaften)*, or (2) properties based on type of contact *(Anschlussarteigenschaften)*.

Differential prosodic properties distinguished between prosodemes themselves. In contrast, the properties based on type of contact did not characterize the prosodemes but the type of contact between the prosodeme and the following phonological element. The distinction between culminative and nonculminative properties was only relevant for the distinctive prosodic properties.

Based on these three major divisions—syllable-counting and mora-counting languages, culminative and non-culminative op-

Table A-1. Prosodic features in Trubetzkoy's *Grundzüge*

	Syllable-counting language	Mora-counting language
Differential properties	Culminative	
	Accent (=stress)	Tone movement
	Nonculminative	
	Intensity (=length)	Tone gemination
Type of contact properties	Nonculminative	
	Close contact	Stød (*Stoss*) close contact

positions, and distinctive prosodic properties and properties based on type of contact—Trubetzkoy's prosodic classification can be represented as in Table A-1.

The Jakobsonian classification of *Fundamentals* distinguished between intersyllabic and intrasyllabic occurrence of prosodic features. The occurrence of a prosodic feature was considered intersyllabic when the crest of one syllable is compared with the crest of another syllable. The occurrence of a prosodic feature was considered intrasyllabic when a portion of a syllable crest was compared to another portion of the same crest or the following slope.

The prosodic features posited by Jakobson consisted of three types: tone, force, and quantity features. In addition to a physical correlate for each of these features, Jakobson also mentioned a "sensation" correlate, represented graphically:

Prosodic feature	Tone	Force	Quantity
Physical correlate	Frequency	Intensity	Time
Sensation correlate	Voice pitch	Voice loudness	Subjective duration

These distinctions yielded the arrangement of features shown in Table A-2.

Table A-2.   Jakobsonian prosodic features in *Fundamentals*

	Intersyllabic	Intrasyllabic
Tone	Tone: high or low level Register	Modulation: high portion of phoneme contrasted with low portion
Force	Stress: louder versus less loud	Stød: loudness of initial portion as contrasted with less loud final portion of phoneme
Quantity	Length: long versus short	Contact: distributional difference in length between vowel and successive consonant

It should be pointed out that the Trubetzkoyan classification and discussion of prosodic features in *Grundzüge* comprised more than forty pages. That of Jakobson in *Fundamentals* was a short survey spanning less than seven pages. An overall comparison of the two systems reveals that the Jakobsonian system appears considerably condensed and unified when compared to that of Trubetzkoy. The following six specific observations can be made.

First, Trubetzkoy based his classification on an analysis of the syllable nucleus rather than of the entire syllable. Based on this analysis, he divided languages into syllable counting and mora counting. Jakobson did not do this. He considered the entire syllable as a base. Within the syllable he distinguished between crest and slope. The slope of the syllable referred to the consonant, the crest to the vowel in a syllable pattern like CVC. Jakobson further maintained that "if the crest contains two or more phonemes, one of them, termed the peak phoneme (or syllabic) is raised over the others by a contrast compact v. diffuse or vowel v. sonorant" (Jakobson and Halle, 1956, p. 21). Even though this initial difference relating to syllable nucleus and syllable between Trubetzkoy and Jakobson appears subtle at first glance, it nevertheless had far-reaching consequences for the entire classification, as shown below.

Second, Jakobson's distinction between intersyllabic prosodic feature (in which the crest of one syllable was compared to the crest of another syllable) and intrasyllabic prosodic feature (in which one portion of the syllable crest was compared to another portion of the same syllable crest or to the following slope) neither corresponds entirely to the Trubetzkoyan dichotomy between differential prosodic properties and properties based on type of contact nor corresponds to the distinction between syllable-counting and mora-counting languages. This lack of correspondence is attributable to Jakobson's intrasyllabic properties, which comprised both a comparison of portions within the same crest and a comparison with the following slope.

Third, tone movement, which for Trubetzkoy occurred in mora-counting languages, in *Fundamentals* was also differentiated within the crest itself. Jakobson renamed "tone movement" *modulation* in *Fundamentals,* thus classing the latter among his intrasyllabic features (together with Trubetzkoy's contact features, that is , the features of stød and close contact). As shown in the Trubetzkoyan classification of Table A-2, tone movement was the equivalent in the mora-counting languages of accent (= stress) in the syllable-counting languages.

Fourth, the Jakobsonian classification also did not distinguish between culminative and nonculˉninative oppositions.[92]
Trubetzkoy, on the other hand, grouped accent and tone movement together as culminative. In contrast, in accordance with his
three prosodic feature types relating to tone, force, and quantity
(see Table A-2), Jakobson classed accent (stress) and modulation
(= tone movement) as intersyllabic and intrasyllabic, respectively. However, accent (stress) for Jakobson was a force feature.
Trubetzkoy thus established the following prosodic rule:

Culminative   → accent (=stress) in syllable-counting languages
                 → tone movement in mora-counting languages

Nonculminative → intensity (length) in syllable-counting languages
                 → tone gemination in mora-counting languages

Jakobson had the following rule:

Tone   → tone, register in an intersyllabic context
                 → modulation (tone movement) in an intrasyllabic
                   context

Force   → stress in an intersyllabic context
                 → stød in an intrasyllabic context

Quantity   → length in an intrasyllabic context
                 → contact in an intrasyllabic context

Fifth, while Trubetzkoy aligned accent (stress) and tone
movement as culminative, Jakobson aligned accent (= stress)
with the correlation of stød, in which "two contiguous fractions of
the stressed phoneme are compared with each other" (Jakobson
and Halle, 1956, p. 24), and where "the initial portion of the
phoneme presents the peak of loudness, whereas in the final portion loudness decreases." For Trubetzkoy stød had been a contact
feature, its physical correlate being "complete or incomplete glottal closure" (1939/1969, p. 197). This is different from the correlate given by Jakobson. However, Trubetzkoy also noted with
respect to stød that acoustically it gives the impression "of two
consecutive sounds, or of a sudden transition within the same
sound from normal voice to a murmur or whisper" (1939/1969,
p. 198). This would represent the equivalent of Jakobson's louder
versus less loud portions. It also represents Jakobson's basis for
considering stress and stød under force features as intersyllabic
and intrasyllabic, respectively.

Sixth, the nonculminative differential properties in the Trubetzkoyan classification comprised the correlation of intensity, the tone feature, and the correlation of gemination. As noted earlier, the tone feature in the Jakobsonian classification was considered as having the sensation correlate of pitch and was realigned with the modulation feature. For the nonculminative differential features, length was the correlate of the intensity and gemination features in the Trubetzkoyan classification. The distinction between intensity and gemination rested on the distinction between syllable-counting and mora-counting languages.

Jakobson, as noted, did not make such a distinction. He therefore was only able to recognize one intersyllabic quantity feature, while intrasyllabically the contact feature—based on the distributional difference in length between vowel and successive consonant—represented a quantity feature. For Trubetzkoy a feature of close contact differentiating between unimpeded, fully developed vowel articulation and interruption of vowel articulation by the following consonant had been a subset of the properties based on type of contact (that is, stød and close contract).

For Jakobson the opposition of contact was based on different distribution of duration between vowel and subsequent consonant. In the case of close contact "the vowel was abridged in favor of the following, arresting consonant, whereas at the open contact the vowel displays its full extent before the consonant starts" (Jakobson and Halle, 1956, p. 24). For Trubetzkoy length was redundant. He described the distinction as follows:

> In the case of close contact the consonant begins at a moment when the articulation of the vowel has not yet passed the peak of its normally rising-falling course, while in the case of the open contact the articulation is fully developed before the onset of the consonant. (1939/1969, p. 199)

The distinction is termed "checked versus unchecked."

It may be mere conjecture that Trubetzkoy introduced the distinction between close and open contact or between checked and unchecked vowels because of difficulties experienced on the morphophonemic level with the archiphoneme concept and neutralization between long and short vowels. The following example illustrates what is meant. In German, where neutralization occurs, the long vowel is found in the position of neutralization. From the point of view of the archiphoneme the long vowel had to be considered as the unmarked member of the opposition long-short vowel. However, the unmarked member of an opposition, at the time of *Grundzüge*, was generally interpreted as "minus the differential property." If length were considered distinctive, the long vowel in the position of neutralization could not have been considered unmarked since it had to be considered "plus the differentiated feature of length." In the case of the distinction between checked and unchecked vowels, on the other hand, an interpretation in accordance with the above general principle was possible. The long vowel occurring in the position of neutralization was also *un*checked and therefore there was no conflict with the interpretation of the *un*marked member as "minus the differentiated property".

As noted earlier, the distinction between checked and unchecked in the above sense has been dropped from the feature framework; *checked* in the Jakobsonian framework was used in a different sense for glottalization.

In contrast to the stød feature, which in the Trubetzkoyan classification could occur only in mora-counting languages and which was reclassified by Jakobson as a force feature, the contact feature in the Jakobsonian classification could occur in both syllable-counting and mora-counting languages.

With respect to the Trubetzkoyan intensity feature, reinterpreted by Jakobson in terms of "intersyllabic length," it may be noted that intensity here was not the same as the Jakobsonian "intensity correlate," which related to the Jakobsonian force feature. However, Trubetzkoy also noted that his intensity feature (=length) rarely occurred by itself. Jakobson noted the same with respect to his intersyllabic force and quantity features (that is, stress and length) in their intersyllabic variety. Jakobson explained that observations "seem to indicate that the prosodic distinctive features utilizing intensity and those utilizing time tend to merge" and that "languages where both length and stress appear as distinctive features are quite exceptional . . . if the stress is distinctive, the latter is mostly supplemented by a redundant length" (Jakobson and Halle, 1956, pp. 24, 25).

Generative phonology contains no definitive study in which the prosodic features have been studied as a set. Wang (1967) observed that tone features were not completely independent from segmental features, having relations to voicing, aspiration, glottalization, and length. He posited a feature contour in which

−*contour* yielded an analysis of five levels of tone by means of the features high, central, and mid; and +*contour* was further subdivided into the feature rising/falling.

In Chomsky and Halle (1968) the following prosodic features were noted: stress; pitch: high, low, elevated, rising, falling, concave; and length. However, they observed that "this subdivision of features is made primarily for purposes of exposition and has little theoretical basis at the present" (p. 300).

As mentioned earlier, Chomsky and Halle did not discuss the prosodic features at all; the above features were merely listed. Prosodic features need further exploration in future phonological studies.

The Major Phonetic Features of the Sound Pattern of English

Major class features
  Sonorant
  Vocalic
  Consonantal
Cavity features
  Coronal
  Anterior
  Tongue-body features
    High
    Low
    Back
  Round
  Distributed
  Covered
  Glottal constrictions
  Secondary apertures
    Nasal
    Lateral
Manner of articulation features
  Continuant
  Release features: instantaneous and delayed
    Primary release
    Secondary release
  Supplementary movements
    Suction
      Velaric suction
      Implosion
    Pressure
      Velaric pressure
      Ejectives
  Tense

As listed in Chomsky and Halle (1968, p. 299).

Source features
  Heightened subglottal pressure
  Voice
  Strident
Prosodic features
  Stress
  Pitch
    High
    Low
    Elevated
    Rising
    Falling
    Concave
  Length

Notes

1. Cf. Horalek (1967).
2. To understand these definitions more fully, the following definitions, also given in *Projet,* are helpful:

   > *Phonological opposition*: a sound difference which serves to differentiate meanings in a given language
   >
   > *Correlational property*: the opposition between the presence and absence of a certain sound feature which differentiates among several pairs of phonological units and which can be thought of independently of individual contrastive pairs
   >
   > *Disjunctive phonological units:* phonological units which are part of the same system but which do not form a correlational pair
   >
   > *Phonological unit*: any member of a phonological opposition
   >
   > *Correlational pair*: each one of the phonological oppositions which form a correlation among themselves

3. Cf. Trubetzkoy's *Die phonologischen Systeme* (1931a, p. 97).
4. However, Trubetzkoy simultaneously and inexplicably restricted the definition of correlation when he continued, "... but the phonemes which are members of these pairs cannot be linked with each other by any other correlative relationships" (p. 97).
5. For example, in *Proposition* we read: "There are two fundamental types of contrast between acoustico-motor images ... the contrast between disjoint images and the contrast between correlative images. The fact that speakers are aware of a correlation between images is solely due to the presence of a series of binary oppositions of the same type in their phonological system. Under these conditions, *linguistic thought* also abstracts a third element (or element of comparison) from the concrete pairs ...." (1929/1962, p. 4; emphasis added). And in *Remarques*: "... the principium divisionis' (classificatory principle) is abstracted by *linguistic consciousness,* and *can be thought of as independent of individual contrastive pairs*" (p. 9; emphasis added).
6. Cf. Bühler (1931, pp. 22–52).
7. We read in *La phonologie actuelle*: "The analysis of different relations between these two types of oppositions (disjunctive

and correlational pairs) and any phonological phenomena pertaining thereto, *makes the discovery of new distinctions and the conceptualization of new notions which require a new terminology possible* . . . (Such terminology) *is absolutely essential since truly new notions and completely unexplored areas are being dealt with"* (1933a, p. 235; emphasis added).

8. Jakobson wrote in *Remarques*: "It would be a *dangerous error of logic* to consider correlations and disjunctive phonemic oppositions on the same level in the analysis of a phonological system and to treat them *without attention to the essential difference* between the two categories and their specific characteristics." And, "Not only are the correlations and the relations between disjunctive phonemes *incommensurable*, but the members of one and the other opposition types do not always coincide as regards their number [do not always occur in equal numbers]" (1929/1962, p. 11; emphasis added).

9. Subsequently this statement was reinterpreted as applying to distinctive features rather than to phonemes, intimating that the above version had been misconstrued. Cf. Jakobson, *Zur Struktur des Phonems* (1939c/1962, p. 301) and *Retrospect* (1962b p. 637).

10. "Phonological unit" *(unité phonologique)* in turn was defined as a "member of any phonological opposition" (cf. text discussion on p. 4 ff.).

11. In *"Tâches à aborder par l'étude d'une système linguistique, du système slave en particulier." TCLP* 1:5–29, 1929.

12. This definition had been given in a monograph on Russian vowels, entitled *Russkie glasnye v kačestvennom i količestvennom otnosenii* (Moscow, 1912), a work which thoroughly impressed a young Jakobson (see Blache, 1978). He wrote: ". . . a work which grew from the quest of Baudouin de Courtenay and followed a trend quite alien to the orthodox disciples of the Moscow linguistic school . . . I was captivated at once by its challenging introductory glosses to the concept of phoneme" (1962b, p. 631).

13. Cf. Trubetzkoy (1936c, p. 10, fn.), where he reiterated the definition of the phoneme given in *Projet*: "The phoneme remains a phonological unit which cannot be analyzed into smaller and simpler phonological units."

14. Trubetzkoy's attitude can be seen from the following quote (1936c, p. 10): ". . . any formula which one accepts for the definition of the phoneme. . . ." In *Grundzüge* Trubetzkoy stated, referring to his *Zur allgemeinen Theorie*: "This writer was at that time not at all interested in the formulation of definitions, but only in the correct application of the phoneme concept. The phoneme concept was used in exactly the same way in the first mentioned phonological articles by the present writer as it is used by him today" (1969, p. 45, fn. 7).

15. See text, p. 4, for a definition of *opposition phonologique*.

16. For a discussion of the differences between the Chomsky and Halle and the Jakobsonian distinctive features, and the relevance of this conflict to speech pathology, see Parker, 1976.

17. In this connection Chomsky and Halle had this to say: "Failure to differentiate sharply between abstract phonological features and concrete phonetic scales has been one of the main reasons for the protracted and essentially fruitless debate concerning the binary character of the Jakobsonian distinctive features" (1968, p. 297, fn. 5).

18. Cf. Trubetzkoy *Die phonologischen Systeme* (1931a, p. 98). For a definition of marked and unmarked, see text p. 35 ff.

19. The development of the concept of morphonology has been treated by L'ubomír Ďurovič (1967).

20. For some controversial data, see Jakobson (1949d/1962, pp. 532–546).

21. Both "mark of correlation" and "correlation mark" are found in English for the German *Korrélationsmerkmal*. Cf. Vachek (1960, 1966).

22. Cf. Trubetzkoy (1933a, p. 236).

23. Ch. Bally had proposed to replace the term *marque* by *caractère différentiel*, which, as it develops, would have been a disservice to posterity. Cf. *Project* (1931, p. 314 fn.).

24. As a native German speaker, I cannot quite subscribe to this conclusion, especially since for Standard German, he would have to consider the voiceless stop as unmarked, and the voiced stop as marked.

25. The terms *langue* and *parole* have been adopted into English as terms of art (cf. Chomsky, 1964, pp. 23, 26). When trans-

lated at all, several equivalents are found, including for *langue* "language system" or "system of language" (cf. Vachek, 1966, pp. 22–26). *Langue* is sometimes also rendered as "linguistic pattern" (cf. Garvin, 1958, pp. vii, 52) and "linguistic system." For *parole* the terms "act of speech" (cf. Garvin, 1958, p. 1), "speech act," "speech event," and "utterance" are also found. Among other terms for *langue* and *parole* used in English are "language" and "speaking" (cf. de Saussure, 1916/1959, pp. 17 ff.); "language" and "speech" (cf. Gardiner, 1932); and "code" and "message" (cf. Jakobson, 1962, p. 465).

26. Jakobson, however, seems to disagree. In *Zur Struktur des Phonems* he has this to say: "The relationship between the study of phonemes or phonology in general and phonetics in no way parallels the relationship between langue and parole but rather the relationship between form and substance" (1939c/1962, p. 310).

27. The term "phonology" as well as the term "phonetics" had, of course, been in use previously. The neogrammarians used the term "phonology" *(Phonologie)* to refer to the historical study of sounds, and "phonetics" *(Phonetik)* to refer to the descriptive study of sounds. For de Saussure, on the other hand, the term *la phonologie* referred to the synchronic study of sounds, whil *le phonetique* referred to the diachronic study of sounds. He stated:

> The physiology of sounds (German, *Laut-* or *Sprachphysiologie*) is often called phonetics *(phonétique, Phonetik)*. To me this name seems inappropriate. Instead I shall use phonology. For phonetics first designated and should continue to designate—the study of the evolution of sounds. Two absolutely distinct disciplines should not be lumped together under the same name. Phonetics is a historical science; it analyzes events and changes, and moves through time. Phonology is outside time, for the articulatory mechanism never changes.
>
> The two studies are distinct but not opposites. Phonetics is a basic part of the science of language; phonology—this bears repeating—is only an auxiliary discipline and belongs exclusively to speaking. (1916/1959, p. 33)

The Saussurian differentiation, as above, however, never became popular. In English, the neogrammarian usage of the word "phonology" had been taken over in the sense of historical study of sound and the "study of the use of sounds in a specific language." The term "phonemics" in English paralleled the Praguian use of the term "phonology." Currently, however, there seems to be a growing preference to use the term "phonology" instead of "phonemics" in English, but in the altered sense of "systematic phonemics." In the past, there has been some reluctance in using the term "phonology" for "phonemics" precisely because of the ambiguous usage of the term as referred to above. Phonology, when used in the sense of phonemics, usually has referred to Prague phonology specifically. (Trubetzkoy himself suggested the term "phonemics" for *Phonologie* in English to avoid any confusion with the prior use of the word in English. (Cf. *Grundzüge*, p. 9.)

28. This statement must be qualified, however, to accommodate the Trubetzkoyan distinction between actually and logically privative oppositions. (Cf. below, p. 60 ff.)

29. The original French term had been *opposition à une seule dimension* for "bilateral" and *opposition à plusieurs dimensions* for "multilateral." Trubetzkoy, in *Essai d'une théorie*, credited K. Bühler for suggesting these. The German *eindimensionale* ("bilateral") and *'mehrdimensionale'* ("multilateral") *Opposition* were used in *Grundzüge*.

30. We read in *Essai d'une théorie* "The differential features of each member of such an opposition are evident with particular clarity because the same relationship between two members is repeated several times in the same system. Thus the phonological analysis of a phoneme as a member of a proportional opposition is made easy and conceiving such a phoneme in terms of the sum of its phonological properties is facilitated" (1936c, p. 11 ff.).

31. We read in *Essai d'une théorie*: "The members of a neutralizable opposition are only different phonemes in those positions where the distinction between them is phonologically relevant. Elsewhere they are merely combinatory variants of a single archiphoneme, that is to say, of a phoneme whose phonological content is reduced to the features which are shared by both members of a given opposition" (1936c, p. 13).

32. Each member of a neutralizable opposition thus has a different phonological content depending on the position in which it occurs in a word. In some environments all its prop-

erties are phonologically relevant, in others some of these properties are not phonologically relevant and therefore lose their distinctiveness. A consequence of this type of "double existence" is that the members of a neutralizable opposition can be analyzed phonologically into "archiphoneme plus specific property," even in those contexts where all its properties are phonologically relevant. On the other hand, where an opposition is constant all properties preserve their phonological value in all positions. As a consequence, the separation of the archiphoneme (that is, the features shared by the two members of a particular opposition) becomes much more difficult (Trubetzkoy, 1936c, p. 13).

33. The original terms used for "linear" and "nonlinear" in *Essai d'une théorie* were *rectiligne* and *curviligne,* respectively.

34. Opposition members here are still phonemes.

35. Cf. Jakobson's *Observations sur le classement phonologique des consones* (1938) and text p. 77 ff.

36. It seems, as evident from the preceding discussion, that the bracket should extend to all three types of oppositions.

37. Occlusives here includes affricates.

38. In part, of course, the distinctions found in the classification based on relations to the entire system were eliminated by the Jakobsonian binary breakthrough itself.

39. For a detached treatise on feature hierarchies, see M.P.R. van den Broecke, *Hierarchies and Rank Orders* (1976).

40. A +/− notation was introduced for the first time, by Jakobson, in 1949 in *On the Identification of Phonemic Entities* (1949c/1962, pp. 418–425) and later in *Notes on the French Phonemic Pattern* (1951/1962, pp. 426–434).

41. It may perhaps be pointed out that binarity also was transferred from opposition to feature.

42. For a definition of the earlier version of correlation, see text discussion p. 3 ff.

43. Trubetzkoy (1939/1969, p. 84) gave the following definition of correlation pair: "By a correlation pair we understand two phonemes that are in a relation of logically privative, proportional, bilateral opposition to each other." And correlation mark "is a phonological property whose presence or absence characterizes a series of correlation pairs."

44. In *Grundzüge* Trubetzkoy recognized close relationships between some of these new correlations. To capture this

phenomenon, he used the term "correlation bundle." Though not explicitly stated in *Grundzüge,* correlation bundles are formed by correlations that are not separated from one another by more than one feature. However, to be considered related, the correlations must have a common parameter that can serve as a classificatory correlate, for example, the different types of work performed by the larynx, or the different types of tensing of the buccal muscles, etc. (The correlation of voice and the correlation of aspiration, for instance, can form a correlation bundle in Sanskrit.) Where this common denominator is lacking, correlations do not form bundles; rather, they are superimposed on one another.

45. To come back to the importance of concrete linguistic evidence for theoretical postulations, it is interesting to note that a systematic search for concrete physical evidence to correlate with the features at a level of theoretical abstraction was first initiated by Jakobson and his colleagues in the late 1940s. In *Preliminaries to Speech Analysis* Jakobson and his collaborators, Fant and Halle, examined acoustic details of a number of languages and reported an inventory of then understood universal features. Despite the fact that few data were available in the perceptual (psychological) domain to verify the perceptual correlates of distinctive features, an effort on their part to indicate such necessarily triggered a great deal of enthusiasm in speech perception (Miller and Nicely, 1955; Wang and Fillmore, 1961; Singh, 1966; Singh and Black 1966; Wickelgren, 1966; Mohr and Wang, 1968; Pols, Van de Kamp, and Plomp, 1969; Singh, Woods, and Becker, 1972; and Danhauer and Singh, 1975).

Van den Broecke (1976) reviewed a series of recent works on distinctive features and speech perception. In these studies, distinctive features have emerged as important parameters in speech perception. Conversely, perceptual correlates have emerged as important cues of distinctive features. As van den Broecke (1976) observed, "if a feature is not distinctive at the perceptual level, it is not distinctive at all" (p. 7), and "for any feature to be meaningful, it must also be verifiable in perception" (p. 85). However, it is also true that to date there exists no adequate framework of the perceptual correlates of distinctive features. Furthermore, as van den Broecke aptly points out, "in no instance is there a one to one relation between articulatory, acoustic, and auditory attributes" of what is defined as a distinctive feature (1976, p. 7). Systematic and simultaneous correspondences between the three types of correlates have always held out an appeal for phonological theory, yet so far have met with less than complete success. Efforts to incorporate perceptual dimensions into phonological theory have so far also not been very successful. The reasons have been summarized by van den Broecke (p. 8 ff.). To date, studies in the perceptual domain of (consonant) features fall into five general categories. Van den Broecke divides these as follows: 1) studies under experimental conditions leading to perceptual confusion, such as acoustic distortion due to white noise and/or various frequency bands of filtering; 2) cross-linguistic perception; 3) recall in short time memory; 4) similarity judgments; and 5) response latencies in similarity judgments. For a complete discussion of the types of studies, types of analysis performed, and features involved, see van den Broecke (1976, pp. 85–120).

46. It may be of interest to note a letter of Trubetzkoy to Jakobson, dated September 19, 1928 (reproduced in *Grundzüge*, 1939/1969, p. 320), where he wrote: "In the meantime I have started working on something else which fascinates me. I have compiled all vocalic systems I knew by heart (thirty-four in all) and tried to compare them . . . I will continue my work on them until I have collected about one hundred languages. The results are extremely strange. All systems can be reduced to a small number of types and can always be respresented by symmetrical diagrams . . . There are some laws about the 'formation of systems' which can be seen without difficulty . . . I believe that the empirical laws discovered in this way will be of great importance . . ."

47. The primacy of the occurrence of the opposition of aperture and the dependency of the opposition of timbre on the presence of the former could account for the fact that in the Trubetzkoyan graphic presentation of vowels we find an inverted vowel triangle or quadrangle compared to the traditional vowel graphs.

48. Recent experiments in vowel perception have substantiated some of Trubetzkoy's early findings on feature primacy and universality. Work in acoustics and perception, for example, has substantiated Trubetzkoy's early claims relating to

the front/back (timbre) dimension and the different degrees of openness (aperture) for vowels of various languages. In attempts to determine the distinctive features of vowels (Pols, Van de Kamp, and Plomp, 1969; Singh and Woods, 1971, 1972; Terbeek and Harshman, 1971; Papcun, 1975), a consistent finding has been the emergence of perceptual/acoustic features of front/back and openness and second formant frequencies, supporting Trubetzkoy's claim for the primacy and basic character of his oppositions of timbre and aperture. These recent findings also indicate that a universal vowel theory is much closer to resolution than a universal consonant theory, in accordance with Trubetzkoy's early vowel-consonant separation. Various studies of production, acoustics, and perception of vowels. For example, work done at the UCLA Phonetics Laboratory points to the universality of the vowel features of aperture, front/back, and rounding.

Recent experiments in vowel perception also show that the front/back dimension carries an inordinantly high amount of weight (Singh, 1966; Grant, 1971; Singh and Woods, 1971).

Regarding the features of intensity and duration, recent analysis of vowel confusions (Verbrugge et al., 1976) have shown that vowel intensity and amplitude play a critical role in English vowel perception.

In summary, there is fairly good concordance in regard to feature universality in the acoustic/perceptual domains of vowels. The difference lies in their priorities (weight). What Trubetzkoy calls "timbre" perceptually is more powerful than any other feature, when verified experimentally (Anglin, 1971; Grant, 1971; Singh and Woods, 1971; Terbeeck and Harshman, 1971). The second feature in rank order is aperture. The other perceptual features such as rounding, length, and intensity are less universal.

49. Although this term sounds almost like Halle's "natural classes," we will see from its application that the two are not really related.

50. It may here be pointed out that Trubetzkoy considered the classification of *Die phonologischen Systeme* supplemental to that given in *Zur allgemeinen Theorie*. He thanked both Jakobson and Sapir for insightful discussions on the subject.

51. However, the distinctive status of the opposition tense/lax is

not established definitively here. The doubts about its distinctiveness relate to the fact that it is frequently redundant. Trubetzkoy wrote (1931a, p. 101): "in case the opposition of tenseness actually occurs as an independent correlation."

52. Trubetzkoy noted that Sapir had called his attention to setting up such an opposition.

53. Cf. Greenberg (1966).

54. Although still found in *Fundamentals,* this last distinction has now been tacitly dropped. The opposition was originally recognized, based on Trubetzkoy's discussion with v. Ginneken. We read in *Die phonologischen Systeme:* ". . . the entire section dealing with the correlation between open and close contact was added after the Prague Phonological Conference. The issue was clarified for me thanks to an interesting and very instructive discussion which I had with Professor J. V. Ginneken at that conference" (p. 102).

55. Apparently Trubetzkoy changed his opinion on the matter subsequently, without it affecting his above classificatory scheme with respect to the oppositions of localization. In *Anleitung zu phonologischen Beschreibungen* he wrote: ". . . proper phonological definition of a phoneme requires accurate classification of all the phonemes in the relevant language. Whether in doing this we use *acoustic* or organogenetic (anatomical) criteria is actually of little import since these terms are only meant to serve as symbols for phonological concepts" (1935/1968, p. 23; emphasis added).

56. In a series of subsequent perceptual experiments involving intricate maneuvering of the acoustic properties of English stop consonants and later other groups of speech sounds, scientists at Haskins Laboratory (Liberman et al., 1967), argued that in the operational hierarchy of speech perception the most crucial reference is speech production (motor theory) rather than acoustics.

57. We read in *Zur allgemeinen Theorie:* "The movements of the lips and tongue result in the alteration of the shape and volume, in particular the length, of the orifice. Different

degrees of timbre correspond to such an alteration acoustically" (1929a/1964, p. 111).

58. A comparative reading of *Preliminaries* and *Fundamentals*
seems to indicate that *Preliminaries* was written in an all-
out effort to classify oppositions with instrumental-acoustic
corollaries, to the neglect of articulatory correlates. In *Fundamentals,* on the other hand, the relationship between
acoustic and articulatory correlates appears more relaxed
and evened out.

59. Jakobson credits Alf Sommerfelt for this observation (1962c,
p. 276).

60. Deleted in proof.

61. It may be interesting to note that Halle (1964, p. 326) distinguishes between four types of constrictiveness: 1) *contact,* in
which opposite parts of the vocal tract touch, as in the case of
the stops; 2) *occlusion,* in which there is an extreme degree
of narrowing, capable of producing turbulence, as in fricative
production; 3) *obstruction,* the next degree of narrowing,
exemplified by articulation of glides, such as /w/ and /j/; and
4) *constriction,* a fourth degree of narrowing as found in
diffuse vowels (e.g., /i/ and /u/). This terminology, however,
largely contradicts existing conventions.

62. Wickelgren (1966) independently investigated Trubetzkoy's
original hypothesis in a series of experiments involving
short-term memory errors of consonants and vowels. Results
of his experiments showed that the disjunctive hypothesis of
consonant and vowel constrictiveness (three degrees of
openness for consonants and three for vowels) is consistent
with the pattern of intrusion errors subjects made in short-
term recall.

63. As to the prosodic features, Chomsky and Halle give a more
straightforward answer when they say that the prosodic features had been omitted from *The Sound Pattern of English*
because their investigation had not been advanced enough
for discussion (see p. 329).

64. The place of articulation parameter has been widely
examined in speech perception. An a posteriori interpretation of perceptual dimensions in multidimensional analysis

has repeatedly shown that consonants in speech perception
are grouped according to a front/back feature. Based on articulatory correlates, this front/back feature directly resem-
bles the Chomsky-Halle anterior/nonanterior feature. In
speech perception, however, there is no recovery of the
coronal/noncoronal features (Danhauer and Singh, 1975;
Singh, Woods, and Becker, 1976).

65.   We read the following with respect to the prosodic units:

> ... the prosodic units ... are rhythmic-melodic units—
> "musical" in the broadest sense of the word. Even from a
> purely phonetic point of view, the "syllable" is basically some-
> thing quite different from a combination of vowels and con-
> sonants. The phonological prosodic unit is, of course, not sim-
> ply identical with the "syllable" (in the phonetic sense). How-
> ever, it always relates to the syllable, because depending on
> the language, it is either a specific segment of the syllable or
> an entire sequence of syllables. It is quite clear that its proper-
> ties cannot be identical with the vocalic and consonantal prop-
> erties discussed above. Since the prosodic unit must be con-
> ceived of as "musical" (rhythmic-melodic), or better, as a seg-
> ment of a "musical unit," it follows that "prosodic properties"
> refer either to the specific marks of each constituent segment
> of a melody (intensity, tone) or to the type of segmentation of
> the melody in the phonation process of human speech.
> (Trubetzkoy, 1939/1969, p. 95)

It may be noted that elsewhere in *Grundzüge* (1939/1969,
p. 170) the wording is not as precise. We simply read that the
prosodic properties belong to the syllables. Notable is the
fact that Trubetzkoy did not define what he meant by syllable. (The same is also true of the terms "syllable peak" for
Trubetzkoy and "syllable crest" by Jakobson. These concepts
have not as yet had any empirical verification, though they
have been used impressionistically for a long time, and
though there has not been a lack of interest or a lack of
investigation. (Cf. Peterson and Lehiste, 1960.)

66.   It may here be noted that in Jakobson and Halle *(Fundamentals)* and in Chomsky and Halle *(Sound Pattern)* only
the obstruction itself, not "overcoming the same," is characteristic for the consonants.

67.   Introduced in that article is the 0 notation to indicate redundancy. It can be replaced by + or − without affecting the
identification of the segment. In *Preliminaries* redundancy
is indicated by brackets.

A ± notation is found in *On the Identification of Phonemic Entities* (Jakobson, 1949c) *Notes on the French Phonemic Pattern* (Jakobson and Lotz, 1951), and *Preliminaries to Speech Analysis* (Jakobson, Fant, and Halle, 1952). In *Notes* the pure features + and − are contrasted with joint features ± (1951/1962, p. 427; also *Preliminaries,* p. 44). Noteworthy is that ± is used by Jakobson to indicate joint presence of two opposed features as well as joint presence of two combined, but separate features. (Cf. *Preliminaries,* ±grave (p. 44) and ±optimal constrictive = +strident (pp. 25, 44).)

68. It should be pointed out here that the term "flat/plain" was used by Trubetzkoy with respect to the consonants, while the term "rounded/unrounded" was used for the vowels. No parallel was drawn.

69. For example, with respect to the resonance features, it is merely stated that "this third class includes . . ." followed by a listing of the features included (Jakobson, Fant, and Halle, 1952, p. 26).

70. It may be pointed out here that the opposition checked/ unchecked, used by Jakobson above as a consonantal feature, in the Trubetzkoyan classification is a vocalic feature in connection with the prosodic opposition of close contact (cf. 1939/1969, p. 116 ff.).

71. Deleted in proof.

72. Deleted in proof.

73. Spectrographic data, however, support the delayed release contention only for initial-position stops. The stops at the medial position may or may not have delayed release and the stops at the final position do not have delayed release (Potter, Kopp, and Green, 1966).

74. In a study by Singh, Woods, and Becker (1972), stridency was rejected as a perceptual feature of English consonants. An a posteriori analysis of perceptual data reveals that the sibilants /s, z, tʃ, dʒ/ cluster together on a dimension (of high perceptual weightings) but the stridents /f, v/ do not join the group. This favors the choice of the feature sibilancy over stridency in speech perception.

75. These were discussed earlier in the text as potentially basic series. Their binary relationship in a language needed to be

substantiated by neutralizability or the presence of second-ary features.

76. Depending on the relationship within a language system, /h/ by Trubetzkoy is considered the "indeterminate consonantal phoneme in general" or it is assigned to a particular localization series, for example, the guttural series or the laryngeal series (the latter, if the language also has a glottal stop; cf. Trubetzkoy, 1939/1969, pp. 138, 140).

77. For describing deviant language behavior and for mapping phonological acquisition of delayed and deviant nature these classifications may prove useful. The basic and the related series may be easier to master than the members of the secondary series. An analysis of developmental data across several languages indicates the order of normal acquisition strategy as: 1) basic series, 2) related series, and 3) secondary series (Singh, 1966).

78. Cf. Ladefoged (1964, pp. 51–54) for the African languages, Effutu and Nkonya.

79. Jakobson criticized Trubetzkoy's table for pharyngeal and nonpharyngeal consonants for Arabic (cf. Jakobson, 1957, p. 516, and Trubetzkoy, 1939/1969, p. 132) for the following reasons: In the Trubetzkoyan classification the nonemphatic consonants /s/ and /z/ lacked an emphatic counterpart, while emphatic /x/ was left with a nonemphatic equivalent and emphatic /χ/ was considered the emphatic equivalent of /g/. Jakobson claims that the opposition between emphatics and nonemphatics should include the pairs /š/ and /ž/ versus /x/ and /χ/. This, however, would leave nonemphatic /g/ without an emphatic counterpart.

80. According to B. Halle, *The Slavonic Languages* (quoted in Kaiser, 1957, p. 303), the degree of rounding may also vary from language to language and thus is not feature dependent in one language. We read (p. 303): "The front vowels of the Slavonic languages are not subject to labialization. This is caused by the fact that the activity of the lips is small as compared to German and French . . . When articulating they are neither rounded nor protruded. Even their articulation of o, u is relatively small. The lips always retain an oval, elliptical shape and are not rounded as, e.g., in French."

81. Similarly, the present framework does not allow for a parallel between palatalization and mid front /e/, since palatalization is represented as +high, /e/ as −high. (See Table 11.)

82. [x^w] here is probably a misprint which should read [h^w].

83. Properties based on the manner of overcoming an obstruction of the third degree refer to the opposition between simple and geminated consonants. Their respective correlates for geminated consonants are longer duration and in most cases also more energic articulation (Trubetzkoy, 1939/1969, p. 161), implying shorter duration and in most cases less energetic articulation for simple, nongeminated consonants. Trubetzkoy here set up what he called the correlation of consonantal gemination. We read: "Geminates are special consonantal phonemes which are distinguished from other consonantal phonemes in that their beginning and end exist phonologically as two separate points, while the beginning and end of all other consonantal phonemes coalesce phonologically into one point" (Trubetzkoy, 1939/1969, p. 162). This distinction was dropped by Jakobson. However, a feature relating to a similar phenomenon with respect to prenasalized consonants is suggested by Chomsky and Halle. See text, p. 150.

84. As mentioned earlier, the parameter of degree of obstruction was found to have important perceptual value in the recall of consonants in short-term memory tasks (Wickelgren, 1966).

85. Trubetzkoy calls this "sonants," not sonorants (1939/1969, p. 141).

86. *Preliminaries* here states (p. 22): ". . . as for the continuant /r/, it is actually a non-syllabic vowel." Also, "the continuant feature may be non-distinctive, as in Japanese."

87. Both Trubetzkoy and Jakobson observed that differentiation by means of the voicing feature is extremely rare for the nasals and liquids.

88. Trubetzkoy had taken the material with respect to Ful from Westerman, *Handbuch der Ful-Sprache,* and Gaden, *Le Poular, dialecte peule du Fouta Sénégalais.* Ladefoged (1968) for Ful (=Fulani) finds the oppositions of prenasalized stops/ stops, laryngealized stops/stops (the former represented by glottal stop plus stop), and nasals/stops with respect to the same place of articulation. Trubetzkoy's above interpretation appears somewhat different: Ladefoged does not find the combination of "nasal + occlusive" in addition to his prenasalized stops. The above Trubetzkoyan seminasalized occlusives thus would appear to correspond to the prenas-

alized stops in the Ladefoged classification. The latter, however, also include what Trubetzkoy considered combinations of "nasal + occlusive."

89. Ladefoged here means prenasalization rather than nasalization.

90. Glides in the Chomsky-Halle classification (1968, p. 303) are divided into two groups: Glides I (/w, y/) and Glides II (/h,ʔ/).

91. Physical here apparently refers to physical data. It may be noted that, in their writings, Chomsky and Halle seem to use the terms "mentalistic" and "psychological reality" in two senses. In one sense the terms pertain to the actual brain mechanism, in the other to intuition or linguistic consciousness. It seems that only the second is mentalistic in the proper sense of the word; the other is far from mentalistic, has nothing to do with linguistic consciousness, and its study is properly scientific.

92. Culminative features were mentioned by Jakobson under configurational features (see Jakobson and Halle, 1956, p. 9) and had a grammatical function.

References

Anglin, M. 1971. Perceptual space of English vowels in word context. Unpublished master's thesis, Howard University, Washington, D.C.

Austerlitz, R. 1964. Review of *A Prague School Reader in Linguistics* (Vachek, 1964). Word 20: 458–465.

Baltaxe, C. 1969. Principles of Phonology (English translation of N.S. Trubetzkoy, *Grundzüge der Phonologie*). University of California Press, Berkeley.

Baltaxe, C. 1969a. The theory of markedness in historical perspective. Presented at the Linguistic Society of America Meeting, summer 1969, Urbana, Ill.

Baskin, W. 1959. A Course in General Linguistics (English translation of F. de Saussure's *Cours de linguistique générale*). In C. C. Bally and A. Sechehaye (eds.), McGraw-Hill, New York.

Baudouin de Courtenay, J. 1895. Versuch einer Theorie phonetischer Alternationen (Ein Kapitel aus der Psychophonetik). Strassburg.

Bell, A. M. 1867. Visible Speech. London.

Birnbaum, H. 1967. Syntagmatische und Paradigmatische Phonologie. In J. Hamm (ed.), Phonologie der Gegenwart, Vorträge und Diskussionen anlässlich der internationalen Phonologie-Tagung in Wien, 30, VIII-3, IX., 1966 (Wiener Slavistisches Jahrbuch, Ergänzungsband 6). Hermann Böhlaus, Graz.

Blache, S. E. 1978. The Acquisition of Distinctive Features. University Park Press, Baltimore.

Bloomfield, L. 1926. A set of postulates for the science of language. Language 2: 153–164. (Repr. in M. Joos, Readings in Linguistics, pp. 26-32. American Council of Learned Societies, Washington, 1957.)

Bloomfield, L. 1933. Language. Holt, Rinehart and Winston, New York.

Bloomfield, L. 1939. Menomini Morphophonemics. Travaux du Cercle linguistique de Prague 8: 105-115. (Repr. in Hockett (ed.), A Leonard Bloomfield Anthology, pp. 351-362 (excerpts). Indiana University Press, Bloomington, 1970.)

Brozović, D. 1967. Some remarks on distinctive features, especially in Standard Serbo-Croatian. In To Honor Roman Jakobson, pp. 412–427. Mouton, The Hague.

The references include the literature cited in the text and the literature used for background research.

Bühler, K. 1931. Phonetik und Phonology. Travaux du Cercle linguistique de Prague 4: 22-53.

Bühler, D. 1934. (2nd ed., 1965). Sprachtheorie. Gustav Fischer Verlag. Stuttgart.

Bühler, K. 1936. Das Strukturmodell der Sprache. Travaux du Cercle linguistique de Prague 6: 3–12.

Cairns, C. E. 1969. Markedness, neutralization, and universal redundancy rules. Language 45: 863–886.

Chomsky, N. 1964. Current Issues in Linguistic Theory. Mouton, The Hague.

Chomsky, N. 1966. Topics in the theory of generative grammar. In T. Sebeok (ed.), Current Trends in Linguistics. 3: Linguistic Theory, pp. 1-58. Indiana University Press, Bloomington.

Chomsky N., and Halle, M. 1968. The Sound Pattern of English. Harper & Row, New York.

Contreras, H. 1969. Simplicity, descriptive adequacy, and binary features. Language 45: 1–9.

Čyževśkyj, D. 1931. Phonologie und Psychologie. Travaux du Cercle linguistique de Prague 4: 3–22.

Danhauer, J. L., and Singh, S. 1975. Multidimensional Speech Perception by the Hearing Impaired. University Park Press, Baltimore.

Diderichsen, P. 1958. The importance of distribution versus other criteria in linguistic analysis. In Proceedings of the Eighth Congress of Linguistics, pp. 156-181. Oslo University Press, Oslo.

Doroszewski, W. 1931. Autour du Phoneme. Travaux du Cercle linguistique de Prague 4: 61–74.

Ďurovič, L. 1967. Das Problem der Morphonologie. In To Honor Roman Jakobson I, pp. 556–569. Mouton, The Hague.

Esper, E. 1968. Mentalism and Objectivism in Linguistics. Elsevier, New York.

Fant, G. 1962. Descriptive analysis of the acoustic aspects of speech. Logos 5: 3–17.

Fant, G. 1967. The nature of distinctive features. In To Honor Roman Jakobson I, pp. 634–643. Mouton, The Hague.

Ferguson, C. 1962. Review of Halle, *The Sound Pattern of Russian* (1959). Language 38: 284–297.

Fischer-Jørgensen, E. 1956. The commutation test and its application to phonemic analysis. In For Roman Jakobson, pp. 140–151. Mouton, The Hague.

Gardiner, A. M. 1932. Speech and Language. Oxford.

Garvin, P. 1953. Review of Jakobson, Fant, and Halle, *Pre-*

liminaries to Speech Analysis. Language 29: 472–482.

Garvin, P. 1958. A Prague Reader on Esthetics, Literary Structure, and Style. 2nd Ed. Institute of Language and Linguistics, Georgetown University, Washington, D.C.

Ginneken, J. van. 1907. Principes de Linguistique Psychologique. Marcel Rivière, Paris.

Grant, M. 1971. INDSCAL Analysis of Hindi and English vowels. Unpublished master's thesis, Howard University, Washington, D. C.

Greenberg, J. 1966. Language Universals. Mouton, The Hague.

Greenberg, J., and Jenkins, J. 1964. Studies in the psychological correlates of the sound system of English. Word 20: 157–177.

Halle, M. 1954. The strategy of phonemics. Word 10: 197–209.

Halle, M. 1957. In defense of the number two. In Studies Presented to Joshua Whatmough on His 60th Birthday, pp. 65-72. Mouton, The Hague.

Halle, M. 1959. The Sound Pattern of Russian. Mouton, The Hague.

Halle, M. 1961. On the role of simplicity in linguistic descriptions. In R. Jakobson (ed.), Proceedings of Symposia in Applied Mathematics, Vol. 12, pp. 89–94. American Mathematical Society, Providence.

Halle, M. 1962. Phonology in generative grammar. Word 18: 54–72. (Repr. in J. A. Fodor and J. Katz (eds.), The Structure of Language: Readings in the Philosophy of Language, pp. 334-352. Prentice-Hall, Englewood Cliffs, N.J.)

Halle, M. 1964. On the bases of phonology. In J. A. Fodor and J. Katz (eds.), The Structure of Language: Readings in the Philosophy of Language, pp. 324-333. Prentice-Hall, Englewood Cliffs, N.J.

Harms, R. 1968. Introduction to Phonological Theory. Prentice-Hall, Englewood Cliffs, N.J.

Harris, J. W. 1969. Sound change in Spanish and the theory of marking. Language 45: 538–553.

Harris, Z. 1941. Review of N. S. Trubetzkoy, *Grundzüge der Phonologie.* Language 17: 345-349.

Harris, Z. 1944. Simultaneous components in phonology. Language 20: 181–205. (Repr. in M. Joos, Readings in Linguistics, pp. 124–139. American Council of Learned Societies, Washington, D.C., 1957.)

Heffner, R. 1950. General Phonetics. University of Wisconsin Press, Madison.

Heny, F. 1967a. Non-binary phonological features. UCLA Working Papers in Phonetics 7: 91–121.

Heny, F. 1967b. Toward the separation of classificatory and phonetic features. UCLA Working Papers in Phonetics 7: 121–125.

Hockett, C. F. 1955. A manual of phonology. International Journal of American Linguistics, Memoir 11. Williams & Wilkins, Baltimore.

Horálek, K. 1964. À propos de la théorie des oppositions binaires. In H. Lundt (ed.), Proceedings of the Ninth International Congress of Linguists, pp. 414–417. Mouton, The Hague.

Horálek, K. 1967. Zum Begriff der phonologischen Korrelation. In J. Hamm (ed.), Phonologie der Gegenwart. Hermann Böhlaus, Graz.

Husserl, E. 1928. Logische Untersuchungen. Max Niemeyer Verlag, Halle, Germany.

Isačenko, A. V. 1956a. Hat sich die Phonologie überlebt? Zeitschrift für Phonetik 9: 311–330.

Isačenko, A. V. 1956b. Sprachwissenschaft und Akustik. Akademie-Verlag, Berlin.

Ivić, M. 1965a. Trends in Linguistics (trans. by Muriel Heppel). Mouton, The Hague.

Ivić, P. 1965b. Roman Jakobson and the growth of phonology. Linguistics 18: 35–79.

Jakobson, R. 1923. O česškom stixe preimuscestvenno u sopostaulenii s russkim. (Repr. in T. Winner (ed.), with English appendices. Brown University Press, Providence, 1969.)

Jakobson, R. 1929. Remarques sur l'évolution phonologique du russe comparée à celle des autres langues slaves. Travaux du Cercle linguistique de Prague 2 (written 1927-1928). (Repr. in R. Jakobson Selected Writings I, pp. 7-117. Mouton, The Hague, 1962.)

Jakobson, R. 1931a. Die Betonung und ihre Rolle in der Wort und Syntagmaphonologie. Travaux du Cercle linguistique de Prague 4. (Repr. in R. Jakobson, Selected Writings I, pp. 117-136. Mouton, The Hague, 1962.)

Jakobson R. 1931b. Z fonologie spisovné slovenštiny. In Studies Presented to Albert Prazak—Slovenska Miscellanea, pp. 155–163, Bratislava. (Repr. as "Phonemic Notes on Standard Slavic," in R. Jakobson, Selected Writings I, pp. 221–230. Mouton, The Hague, 1962.)

Jakobson, R. 1932a. Zur Struktur des russischen Verbums. Charisteria Guilelmo Mathesio oblata, Prague. (Repr. in J.

Vachek (ed.), A Prague School Reader in Linguistics, pp. 347–359. Indiana University Press, Bloomington, 1966.)

Jakobson, R. 1932b. Phoneme and phonology. In the Second Supplementary Volume to the Czech Encyclopedia, Ottův slovník naučný, Prague. (Repr. in R. Jakobson, Selected Writings I, pp. 231–234. Mouton, The Hague, 1962.)

Jakobson, R. 1936a. Beitrag zur allgemeinen Kasuslehre. Travaux du Cercle linguistique de Prague 6: 240–288. (Repr. in E. P. Hamp et al. (eds.), Readings in Linguistics II, pp. 51-89. The University of Chicago Press, Chicago, 1966.)

Jakobson, R. 1936b. Über die Beschaffenheit der prosodischen Gegensätze. In Melanges de Linguistique et de Philosophie Offerts à J. van Ginneken (1937), Paris. (Repr. in R. Jakobson, Selected Writings I, pp. 254-261. Mouton, The Hague, 1962.)

Jakobson, R. 1937. On ancient Greek prosody (publ. in Polish). Studies presented to Kazimierz Woyzcicki-z zagadnien poetyki VI, Wilno. (Repr. in R. Jakobson, Selected Writings I, pp. 262–272. Mouton, The Hague, 1962.)

Jakobson, R. 1938. Observations sur le classement phonologique des consonnes. In Proceedings of the Third International Congress of Phonetic Sciences (1939), Geneva. (Repr. in R. Jakobson, Selected Writings I, pp. 272-280. Mouton, The Hague, 1962.)

Jakobson, R. 1939a. Nécrologie Nikolaj Serjeevič Trubetzkoy. Acta Linguistica 1: 64–76. (Repr. in T. E. Sebeok (ed.), Portraits of Linguists, pp. 526–543. Indiana University Press, Bloomington, 1966.)

Jakobson, R. 1939b. Un manuel de phonologie générale. Acta Linguistica I. (Repr. in R. Jakobson, Selected Writings I, pp. 311–317. Mouton, The Hague, 1962.)

Jakobson, R. 1939c. Zur Struktur des Phonems (based on two lectures at the University of Copenhagen). (Repr. in R. Jakobson, Selected Writings I, pp. 280-311. Mouton, The Hague, 1962.)

Jakobson, R. 1942. Kindersprache, Aphasie und allgemeine Lautgesetze. Originally published in *Sprakvetenskapliga Sallskapets Forhandlingar,* Uppsala. (Repr. in R. Jakobson, Selected Writings I, pp. 329–396. Mouton, The Hague, 1962d.)

Jakobson, R. 1949a. Les lois phoniques du langage enfantin et leur place dans la phonologie générale. (Prepared for the Fifth International Congress of Linguists, Brussels, 1939.) Published as a supplement to Cantineau's translation of N. S. Trubetzkoy, Grundzüge der Phonologie: Principes de Phonologie, Paris.

(Repr. in R. Jakobson, Selected Writings I, pp. 317–329. Mouton, The Hague, 1962.)

Jakobson, R. 1949b. Notes autobiographiques de N. S. Trubetzkoy. In Cantineau's translation of N. S. Trubetzkoy, Grundzüge der Phonologie: Principes de Phonologie, pp. xv-xxix, Paris. (Also in the supplement to Baltaxe's English translation, Principles of Phonology, pp. 309–323. University of California Press, Berkeley, 1969.)

Jakobson, R. 1949c. On the identification of phonemic entities. Travaux du Cercle linguistique de Copenhague 5: 205–213. (Repr. in R. Jakobson, Selected Writings I, pp. 418–426. Mouton, the Hague, 1962.)

Jakobson, R. 1949d. Why "Mama" and "Papa"? (Originally published in French.) (Repr. in R. Jakobson, Selected Writings I, pp. 538–545. Mouton, The Hague, 1962.)

Jakobson, R. 1951. For the correct presentation of phonemic problems. Symposium V, Syracuse. (Repr. in R. Jakobson, Selected Writings I, pp. 435-443. Mouton, The Hague, 1962.)

Jakobson, R. 1956. Serge Karcevski. In Cahiers Ferdinand de Saussure XIV: 9-13. (Repr. in T. E. Sebeok (ed.), Portraits of Linguists, pp. 493-497. Indiana University Press, Bloomington, 1966.)

Jakobson, R. 1957. Mufaxxama, the 'emphatic' phonemes in Arabic. In Studies Presented to Joshua Whatmough on His 60th Birthday, pp. 105–115. Mouton, The Hague. (Repr. in R. Jakobson, Selected Writings I, pp. 510–522. Mouton, The Hague, 1962.)

Jakobson, R. 1961. The phonemic concept of distinctive features. Proceedings of the Fourth International Congress of Phonetic Sciences, pp. 440–455. Mouton, The Hague.

Jakobson, R. 1962a. Efforts toward a means-ends model in language in interwar continental linguistics. In Trends in European and American Linguistics 1930–1960, II, Utrecht. (Repr. in J. Vachek (ed.), A Prague School Reader in Linguistics, pp. 481–485. Indiana University Press, Bloomington, 1964.)

Jakobson, R. 1962b. Retrospect. In R. Jakobson, Selected Writings I, pp. 629–659. Mouton, The Hague, 1962.

Jakobson, R. 1962c. Selected Writings I. Mouton, The Hague.

Jakobson, R. 1966. The role of phonic elements in speech perception. 18th International Congress of Psychology, Symposium 23:

Models of Speech Perception. (Repr. by the Salk Institute for Biological Studies, San Diego, Cal., 12 pp. Repr. with Russian abstract in Zeitschrift für Phonetik, Sprachwissenschaft und Kommunikationsforschung, 21: 9–20, 1968.)

Jakobson, R. 1971. A bibliography of his writing. In C. H. van Schooneveld (ed.), Janua Linguarum, Studia Memoriae Nicolai Van Wijk dedicata. Mouton, The Hague.

Jakobson, R. (ed.). 1975. N. S. Trubetzkoy's Letters and Notes. Mouton, The Hague.

Jakobson, R., Cherry, E., and Halle, M. 1953. Toward a logical description of languages in their phonemic aspect. Language 29. (Repr. in R. Jakobson, Selected Writings, I, pp. 449–464. Mouton, The Hague, 1962.)

Jakobson, R., Fant, G., and Halle, M. 1952. Preliminaries to Speech Analysis. MIT Press, Cambridge, Mass.

Jakobson, R., and Halle, M. 1956. Fundamentals of Language. Mouton, The Hague.

Jakobson, R., and Halle, M. 1963. Tenseness and Laxness. Supplement to *Preliminaries to Speech Analysis,* pp. 57–61, 3rd Ed. MIT Press, Cambridge, Mass.

Jakobson, R., Karcevskij, S., and Trubetzkoy, N. 1928. Proposition au Premier Congrès International de Linguistes (Quelles sont les méthodes les mieux appropriées à un exposé complèt et pratique de la phonologie d'une langue quelconque?). Actes du Premier Congrès International de Linguistes du 10–15 avril, 1928. (Repr. in R. Jakobson, Selected Writings I, pp. 3–6. Mouton, The Hague, 1962.)

Jakobson, R., and Lotz, J. 1949. Notes on the French Phonemic Pattern. Word 5: 151–158. (Repr. in R. Jakobson, Selected Writings I, pp. 426–435. Mouton, The Hague, 1962.)

Kaiser, L. (ed.). 1957. A Manual of Phonetics. North-Holland, Amsterdam.

Kim, C. 1966. On the linguistic specification of speech. Unpublished doctoral dissertation, University of California, Los Angeles.

Klatt, D. 1968. Structure of confusions in short term memory between English consonants. J. Acoust. Soc. Am. 44: 401–407.

Kurylowicz, J. 1960. Esquisses Linguistiques. Wroclaw, Krakow.

Kurylowicz, J. 1967. Phonologie und Morphonologie. In J. Hamm (ed.), Phonologie der Gegenwart. Hermann Böhlaus, Graz.

Ladefoged, P. 1964. A Phonetic Study of West African Languages. West African Monographs 1. Cambridge University Press, Cambridge. (2nd Ed., 1968.)

Ladefoged, P. 1970. The Phonetic Framework of Generative Phonology. University of California, Los Angeles. (Mimeograph.)

Ladefoged, P. 1972. Phonological features and their phonetic correlates. J. Int. Phonet. Assoc. 2: 2–12.

Ladefoged, P. 1977. The abyss between phonetics and phonology. Paper presented at the 13th Annual Meeting of the Chicago Linguistic Society, Chicago, spring 1977.

Ladefoged, P., and Vennemann, T. 1973. Phonetic features and phonological features. Lingua 32: 61–74.

Lakoff, G. 1965. Markedness in Phonology. (Mimeograph).

LeRoy, M. 1967. Main Trends in Modern Linguistics (trans. by Glenville Price). University of California Press, Berkeley.

Liberman, A. M., Cooper, F. S., Shankweiler, D. P., and Studdert-Kennedy, M. 1967. Perception of the speech code. In E. E. David and P. B. Denes (eds.), Human Communication: A Unified Vew, pp. 13–51. McGraw-Hill, New York.

Lightner, T. 1965. Russian Phonology. MIT Press, Cambridge, Mass.

Lindau, M. 1975. Features for vowels. UCLA Working Papers in Phonetics 30.

Malmberg, B. 1963. Structural Linguistics and Human Communication. Springer Verlag, Berlin.

Marouzeau, J. 1933. Lexique de la Terminologie Linguistique. Paris.

Martinet, A. 1936. Neutralisation et archiphoneme. Travaux du Cercle linguistique de Prague 6: 46–57.

Martinet, A. 1949. Phonology as Functional Phonetics. Basil Blackwell, Oxford.

Martinet, A. 1962. A Functional View of Language. Oxford University Press, London.

Martinet, A. 1964. Elements of General Linguistics (English translation of E. Palmer's *Elements de linguistique generale,* 1960). Faber and Faber, London.

McCawley, Jr. 1967. Le rôle d'un système des traits phonologiques dans une théorie du langage. Langages 7: 112–123.

Miller, G. A., and Nicely, P. A. 1955. An analysis of perceptual confusions among some English consonants. J. Acoust. Soc. Am. 27: 338–352.

Mohr, B., and Wang, W. 1968. Perceptual distance and the specification of phonological features. Phonetica 18: 31–45.

Newmann, P. 1968. The reality of the morphophoneme. Language 44: 507–516.

Otto, E. 1959. Stand und Aufgabe der allgemeinen Sprachwissenschaft. Walter de Gruyter, Berlin.

Papcun, G. 1975. How can vowel systems differ? J. Acoust. Soc. Am. 58: S119.

Parker, F. 1976. Distinctive features in speech pathology: Phonology or phonetics? J. Speech Hear. Disord. 41: 23–39.

Peterson, G. E., and Barney, H. I. 1952. Control methods used in the study of vowels. J. Acoust. Soc. Am. 24: 175–184.

Peterson, G., and Lehiste, I. 1960. Duration of syllable nuclei in English. J. Acoust. Soc. Am. 32: 693–703.

Pols, L., Van de Kamp, L., and Plomy, R. 1969. Perceptual and physical space of vowel sounds. J. Acoust. Soc. Am. 46: 458–467.

Postal, P. 1968. Aspects of Phonological Theory. Harper & Row, New York.

Potter, R., Kopp, G., and Green, H. 1966. Visible Speech. 2nd Ed. Dover, New York.

Projet de terminologie phonologique standardisée. 1931. Travaux du Cercle linguistique de Prague 4.

Romportl, M. 1963. Zur akustischen Struktur der Distinctiven Merkmale. Zeitschrift für Phonetik 16: 191–198.

Sapir, E. 1925. Sound patterns of language. Language 1: 37–51. (Repr. in M. Joos, Readings in Linguistics, pp. 19–25. American Council of Learned Societies, Washington, D. C., 1957.)

Sapir, E. 1933. The psychological reality of phonemes. Originally published in French. (Repr. in Selected Writings of Edward Sapir in Language, Culture, and Personality, pp. 225–250. University of California Press, Berkeley, 1949.)

de Saussure, F. 1916. Cours de linguistique générale, Paris. (Baskin trans.: A Course in General Lingusitics, 1959.)

Shane, S. 1968. On the non-uniqueness of phonological representations. Language 44: 709–717.

Shepard, R. N. 1972. Psychological representation of speech sounds. In E. E. David, Jr., and P. B. Denes (eds.), Human

Communications: A Unified View, pp. 67–113. McGraw-Hill, New York.

Sievers, E. 1901. Grundzüge der Phonetik. Breitkopf und Hartel, Leipzig.

Singh, S. 1966. Cross-language study of perceptual confusion of plosive phonemes in two conditions of distortions. J. Acoust. Soc. Am. 40: 635–656.

Singh, S. 1974. A step toward a theory of speech perception. Reprints of the Communication Seminar, August, Stockholm.

Singh, S. 1975. Distinctive Features: Theory and Validation. University Park Press, Baltimore.

Singh, S., and Black, J. W. 1966. Study of twenty-six intervocalic consonants as spoken and recognized by four languages groups. J. Acoust. Soc. Am. 39: 372–387.

Singh, S., and Woods, D. R. 1971. Perceptual structure of 12 American English vowels. J. Acoust. Soc. Am. 49: 1861–1866.

Singh, S., and Woods, D. R. 1972. Implication of the perception of similarities for phonetic theory. In A. Rigualt and R. Carbonneau (eds.), Proceedings of the 7th International Congress of Phonetic Sciences, pp. 608–612. Mouton, The Hague.

Singh, S., Woods, D. R., and Becker, G. M. 1972. Perceptual structure of 22 prevocalic English consonants. J. Acoust. Soc. Am. 52: 1698–1713.

Stankiewicz, E. 1967. Opposition and hierarchy in morphophonemic alternation. In To Honor Roman Jakobson, Essays on the Occasion of His Seventieth Birthday III, pp. 1895–1904. Mouton, The Hague.

Stanley, R. 1967. Redundancy rules in phonology. Language 43: 393–437.

Sweet, H. 1906. A Primer of Phonetics. Henry Frowde, Oxford.

Terbeek, D., and Harshman, R. 1971. Crosslanguage differences in the perception of natural vowel sounds. UCLA Working Papers in Phonetics 19: 26–38.

Thèses presentées au premier Congrès des philologues slaves. 1929. Travaux du Cercle linguistique de Prague 1: 5–29. (Repr. in J. Vachek (ed.), A Prague School Reader in Linguistics, pp. 33–58. Indiana University Press, Bloomington, 1964.)

Trnka, B. 1936. General Laws of Phonemic Combinations. Travaux du Cercle linguistique de Prague 6: 57–62.

Trnka, B., et al. 1964. Prague structural linguistics. In J. Vachek (ed.), A Prague School Reader in Linguistics, pp. 468–480. Indiana University Press, Bloomington.

Trubetzkoy, N. S. 1929a. Zur allgemeinen Theorie der phonologischen Vokalsysteme. Travaux du Cercle linguistique de Prague 1: 39–67. (Repr. in J. Vachek (ed.), A Prague School Reader in Linguistics, pp. 108–142. Indiana University Press, Bloomington, 1964.)

Trubetzkoy, N. S. 1929b. Sur la "morphonologie," Travaux du Cercle linguistique de Prague 1: 85–88. (Repr. in J. Vachek, A Prague School Reader in Linguistics, pp. 183–186. Indiana University Press, Bloomington, 1964.)

Trubetzkoy, N. S. 1929c. Polabische Studien. Akademie der Wissenschaften in Wien, Philos.-hist. Kl., Bd. 211, Abh. 4.

Trubetzkoy, N. S. 1931a. Die phonologischen Systeme. Travaux du Cercle linguistique de Prague 4: 96–116.

Trubetzkoy, N. S. 1931b. Gedanken über die Morphonologie. Travaux du Cercle linguistique de Prague 4: 160–163. (Repr. in Appendix II, Baltaxe's English translation of N.S. Trubetzkoy, Grundzüge der Phonologie: Principles of Phonologie, pp. 305–308. University of California Press, Berkeley, 1969.)

Trubetzkoy, N. S. 1931c. Phonologie und Sprachgeographie. Travaux du Cercle linguistique de Prague 4: 228–234. (Repr. in Appendix I, Baltaxe's English translation of N.S. Trubetzkoy, Grundzüge der Phonologie: Principles of Phonology, pp. 298–304. University of California Press, Berkeley, 1969.)

Trubetzkoy, N.S. 1931d. Principes de transcription phonologique. Travaux du Cercle linguistique de Prague 4: 323–326.

Trubetzkoy, N. S. 1931e. Die Konsonantensysteme der ostkaukasischen Sprachen. Caucasica, fasc. 8: 1–52.

Trubetzkoy, N. S. 1933a. La phonologie actuelle. Journal de Psychologie 30: 227–246.

Trubetzkoy, N. S. 1933b. Les systemes phonologiques envisagés en eux-mêmes et dans leurs rapports avec la structure générale de la langue. Actes du deuxième congrès international de linguistes, Genève, 25–29 aout, 1931, Paris, pp. 109–113, 120–125.

Trubetzkoy, N. S. 1933c. Charakter and Methode der systematischen Darstellung einer gegebenen Sprache. Proceedings of the International Congress of Phonetic Sciences, Amsterdam, July 3–8, 1932, (Archives néerlandaises de phonétique expérimentale VIII-IX, 1933), pp. 18–22.

Trubetzkoy, N. S. 1934. Das morphonologische Systeme der russischen Sprache. Travaux du Cercle linguistique de Prague 52.

Trubetzkoy, N. S. 1935. Anleitung zu phonologischen Beschreibungen. Association internationale pour les études phonologiques; publ. by The Prague Linguistique Circle, Brno, 32 pp.; trans. by L. Murray: Introduction to the Principles of Phonological Descriptions, Martinus Nijhoff, The Hague, 1968.

Trubetzkoy, N. S. 1936a. Die phonologischen Grenzsignale. Proceedings of the Second International Congress of Phonetic Sciences, London, July 22−26, 1935, Cambridge, 45−49.

Trubetzkoy, N. S. 1936b. Die Aufhebung der phonologischen Gegensätze. Travaux du Cercle linguistique de Prague 6: 29−45. (Repr. in J. Vachek, A Prague School Reader in Linguistics, pp. 185−205. Indiana University Press, Bloomington, 1964.)

Trubetzkoy, N. S. 1936c. Essai d'une théorie des oppositions phonologiques. Journal de Psychologie 33: 5−18.

Trubetzkoy, N. S. 1936d. Die phonologischen Grundlagen der sogenannten 'Quantität' in den verschiedenen Sprachen. Scritti in onore di Alfredo Trombetti, Milan, pp. 155−176.

Trubetzkoy, N. S. 1936e. Die Quantität als phonologisches Problem. IVè Congrès international de linguistes, Copenhague, 1936, Resumés de communications, 104−105.

Trubetzkoy, N. S. 1937. Über eine neue Kritik des Phonembegriffs. Archiv für die vergleichende. Phonetik 1: 129−153.

Trubetzkoy, N. S. 1938. Actes du Quatrième congrès international de linguistes ténue à Copenhague du 27 août au 1er septembre 1936, Copenhagen, 117−122.

Trubetzkoy, N. S. 1939. Grundzüge der Phonologie. Travaux du Cercle linguistique de Prague 7. (English trans. by C. Baltaxe: Principles of Phonology. University of California Press, Berkeley, 1969.)

Twaddell, F. 1935. On defining the phoneme. Language Monograph 16. (Repr. in M. Joos, Readings in Linguistics, pp. 55−81. American Council of Learned Societies, Washington, D. C., 1957.)

Ułaszyn, H. 1931. Laut, Phonema, Morphonema. Travaux du Cercle linguistique de Prague 4: 53−61.

Ułasyn, H. 1927. Prace Filolojiczne 12: 60.

Vachek, J. 1936. Phonemes and phonological units. Travaux du Cercle linguistique de Prague 4: 235−240. (Repr. in J. Vachek, A Prague School Reader in Linguistics, pp. 143−150. Indiana University Press, Bloomington, 1964.)

Vachek, J. 1960. Dictionnaire de linguistique de l'école de Prague. Comité International Permanent Linguistique, Utrecht.

Vachek, J. 1964. A Prague School Reader in Linguistics. Indiana University Press, Bloomington.

Vachek, J. 1966. The Linguistic School of Prague. Indiana University Press, Bloomington.

Vachek, J. 1977. Review of N. S. Trubetzkoy's Letters and Notes. Prepared for publication by Roman Jakobson. Language 53: 424.

van den Broecke, M. P. R. 1976. Hierarchies and Rank Orders in Distinctive Features. Assen, van Gorcum, Holland.

van den Broecke, M. P. R., and Goldstein, L. 1977. Consonant features in speech errors. Paper presented at the Third Meeting of Acoustic Society of America, State College, Penn., spring.

Vennemann, T. 1970. The high German consonant shift in the perspective of markedness theory. In R. P. Stockwell (ed.), Historical Linguistics in the Perspective of Transformational Theory. Proceedings of the 1969 Conference at UCLA. Indiana University Press, Bloomington.

Vennemann, T., and Ladefoged, P. 1973. Phonetic features and phonological features. Lingua 32: 61–74.

Verbrugge, R. R., Strange, W., Shankweiler, D. P., and Edman, P. R. 1976. What information enables a listener to map a talker's vowel space? J. Acoust. Soc. Am. 60: 198–212.

Walsh, H. 1974. On certain inadequacies of distinctive feature systems. J. Speech. Hear. Disord. 39: 32–43.

Wang, W. S. 1967. Phonological features of tone. Int. J. Am. Ling. 33: 93–105.

Wang, W. S. 1968. Vowel features, paired variables, and the English vowel shift. Language 44: 695–709.

Wang, M., and Bilger, R. C. 1973. Consonant confusions in noise: A study of perceptual features. J. Acoust. Soc. Am. 54: 1248–1266.

Wang, W., and Fillmore, C. 1961. Intrinsic cues in consonant perception. J. Speech Hear. Res. 4: 130–136.

Wells, R. S. 1947. De Saussure's system of linguistics. Word 3: 1–31. (Repr. in M. Joos (ed.), Readings in Linguistics, pp. 1–18. American Council of Learned Societies, Washington, D.C., 1957.

Wickelgren, W. A. 1966. Distinctive features and errors in short-term memory for English consonants. J. Acoust. Soc. Am. 39: 388–398.

Wilson, R. 1966. A criticism of distinctive features. J. Ling. 2: 195–206.

Index

Acoustic, interpretations of the term, 80

Acoustic correlates for vowels, 95-108

Acoustic impressions related to consonant and vowel oppositions, 82

Actual variants of proportional oppositions, 59-60, 66

Acute consonants and grave consonants, distinction between, 79-80, 81, 85-87

Affricates, bases for differentiation of, 113-114, 115, 116-117

Alphabetic symbols, 16-17

Aperture, oppositions of, for vowels, 69, 70-72, 73, 95-108

Apicals
and palatals, opposition between, 124
and retroflexes, opposition between, 124
and sibilants, binary relations between, 109

Archiphoneme
and morphophoneme, relationship between, 30-35
representative of, 44
symbol for, 43-44

Archiphoneme concept
addition of neutralization to, 23-30
changes in, 20-23
in Prague phonology, 19-35

Archi-segment in feature framework, 17

Archi-unit in feature complex, 17

Articulation
point of, parameter for, binary analysis of, 77-85
position of, oppositions based on, for vowels, 69-72, 73, 95-108
primary and secondary, relationship between, 119-124, 125, 132, 136
secondary, features in, 127

Aspiration feature, 155-156

Back consonants and front consonants, distinction between, 79-80

Baudouin de Courtenay on approaches to sound study, 47

Bilateral oppositions, 51-52, 53-54
and binary oppositions, distinction between, 54-55
divisions of, 57
and multilateral oppositions, distinction between, 55-56
and neutralization, 25-27

Binary analysis of point of articulation parameter, 77-85

Binary classification of vowels, 98-99

Binary distinctive feature system, exploration of, 68-90

Binary oppositions, 62-65, 67-68
and bilateral oppositions, distinction between, 54-55
and gradual oppositions, distinction between, 63
of vowels, 71-72

Bloomfield, L., on morphophonemes, 34-35

Boundary in feature framework, 17

Chomsky, N.
on alphabetic symbols, 16-17
on application of markedness to timbre and tonality features, 104
on distinctive features, 15-16
feature classification system of, 17-19, 86-87, 134-138, 151-156

211

and rounding in vowels, relation between, 131-138
Labialized velars, characterization of, 135
Labials
and rounding in vowels, relation between 131-138
velarized, characterization of, 135
Labiovelars
classification of, 134-135
and velars
binary relations between, 109-110
opposition between, 124
Laxness feature, 146-148
Linear oppositions, 52
Liquids
classification of, 144, 158
definition of, 83
Localization features for consonants, 109-138
basic series of, 109-111, 124-126
related series of, 111-119, 124-126
secondary series of, 119-126
Logical variants of proportional oppositions, 59-60, 66

Markedness
applicaton of, to timbre and tonality features, 104
concept of
current, 45-47
in generative phonology, 35-47
origin of, 39-45
in Prague phonology, 35-47
origin of term, 38-39
Martinet, A., on archiphoneme and neutralization, 29-30
McCawley, Jr., on rounding and pharyngealization, 125-126
Mellow consonants and strident consonants, distinction between, 83-84
Mellowness feature in classification of consonants, 112-117

Melody, oppositions of, for vowels, 74
Monte Negran dialects, vowel system of, analysis of, 98-99, 102
Mora-counting languages, 171, 172
Mora, definition of, 171
Morphophoneme
and archiphoneme, relationship between, 30-35
concept of, in Prague phonology, 30-35
Morphophonology, definition of, 31-32
Multilateral oppositions, 51-52, 53-54
and bilateral oppositions, distinction between, 55-56

Nasal consonants and oral consonants, distinction between, 82
Nasalization, analysis of, 148-151
Natural feature classes, 72-77
Naturalness
as criteria for basic consonant classes, 109
and markedness, 41-42, 46
Neutralizable oppositions, 52, 53
phonological content of, 185-186
Neutralization
addition of, to archiphoneme concept, 23-30
concept of, in Prague phonology, 23-30
as criteria for related series of consonants, 109
and markedness, 44-45
Nonlinear oppositions, 52-53
Nuclei, syllable, definition and composition of, 171

Obstruction
of first degree, properties for consonants based on overcoming of, 138-140